ENOUGH

ENOUGH

Climbing Toward a True Self on Mount Everest

MELISSA ARNOT REID

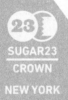

SUGAR23

CROWN

NEW YORK

Published in the United States by Crown, an imprint of the Crown Publishing Group,
a division of Penguin Random House LLC, New York.
crownpublishing.com

CROWN and the Crown colophon are registered trademarks of
Penguin Random House LLC.

Sugar23 and the Sugar23 logo are registered trademarks of Sugar23, Inc.

Map by Nick Springer, copyright © 2025 Springer Cartographics

Library of Congress Cataloging-in-Publication Data
Names: Reid, Melissa Arnot, author.
Title: Enough : climbing toward a true self on Mount Everest / Melissa Arnot Reid.
Description: First edition. | New York : Crown Publishing, [2025]
Identifiers: LCCN 2024042010 (print) | LCCN 2024042011 (ebook) |
ISBN 9780593594087 (hardcover) | ISBN 9780593594094 (ebook)
Subjects: LCSH: Reid, Melissa Arnot. | Women mountaineers—United States—
Biography. | Mountaineers—United States--Biography. | Mountaineering—Psychological
aspects. | Self-actualization (Psychology) | Everest, Mount (China and Nepal)
Classification: LCC GV199.92.R446 A3 2025 (print) | LCC GV199.92.R446 (ebook) |
DDC 796.522092 [B]—dc23/eng/20250115
LC record available at https://lccn.loc.gov/2024042010
LC ebook record available at https://lccn.loc.gov/2024042011

Hardcover ISBN 978-0-593-59408-7
Ebook ISBN 978-0-593-59409-4

Printed in the United States of America on acid-free paper

Editor: Kevin Doughten
Associate editor: Amy Li
Editorial assistant: Jess Scott
Production editor: Sohayla Farman
Text designer: Amani Shakrah
Production manager: Dustin Amick
Copy editor: Alison Kerr Miller
Proofreaders: JoAnna Kremer, Judy Kiviat, and Eldes Tran
Publicist: Stacey Stein
Marketer: Mason Eng

1 2 3 4 5 6 7 8 9

First Edition

The authorized representative in the EU for product safety and compliance is
Penguin Random House ireland, Morrison Chambers, 32 Nassau Street,
Dublin D02 YH68, Ireland, https://eu-contact.penguin.ie.

For Kaia and Judah.
You are, and will always be, enough.
And for Tyler, for reminding me that I am too.

CONTENTS

IV

V

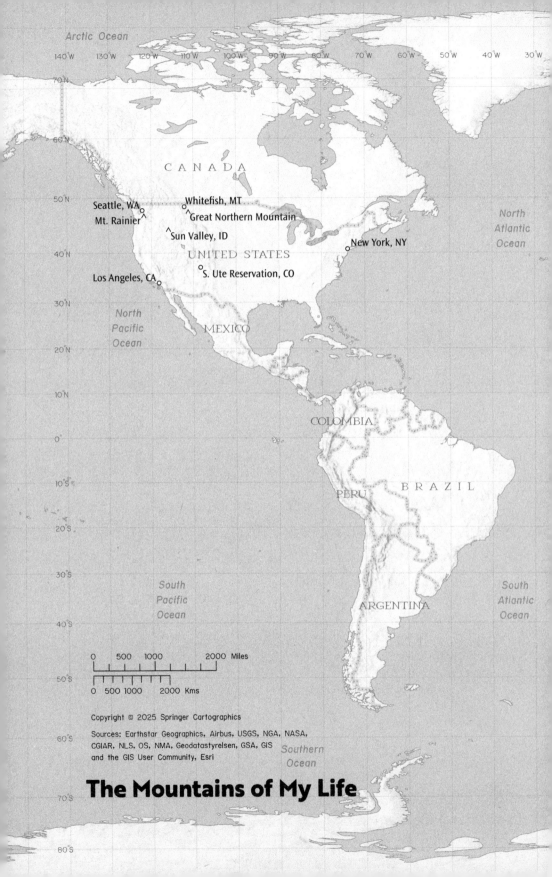

Arctic Ocean

CANADA

Seattle, WA
Mt. Rainier

Whitefish, MT
Great Northern Mountain

Sun Valley, ID

UNITED STATES

New York, NY

North
Atlantic
Ocean

Los Angeles, CA

S. Ute Reservation, CO

North
Pacific
Ocean

MEXICO

COLOMBIA

PERU

BRAZIL

South
Pacific
Ocean

ARGENTINA

South
Atlantic
Ocean

0   500   1000   2000 Miles

0 500 1000   2000 Kms

Copyright © 2025 Springer Cartographics

Sources: Earthstar Geographics, Airbus, USGS, NGA, NASA,
CGIAR, NLS, OS, NMA, Geodatastyrelsen, GSA, GIS
and the GIS User Community, Esri

Southern
Ocean

The Mountains of My Life

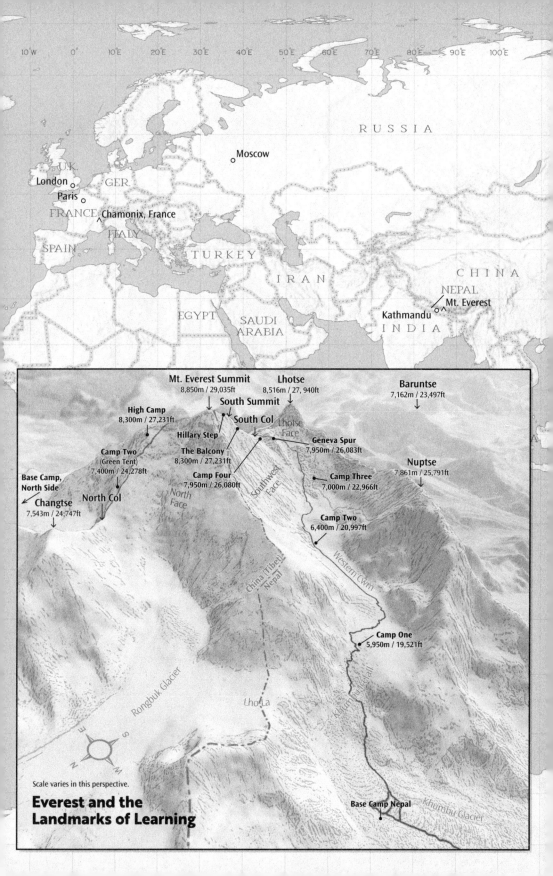

10°W 0° 10°E 20°E 30°E 40°E 50°E 60°E 70°E 80°E 90°E 100°E

RUSSIA

Moscow

U.K.
London
Paris   GER.
FRANCE   Chamonix, France
ITALY
SPAIN   TURKEY
IRAN   CHINA
NEPAL
EGYPT   SAUDI   Mt. Everest
ARABIA   Kathmandu   INDIA

Mt. Everest Summit
8,850m / 29,035ft

Lhotse
8,516m / 27, 940ft

High Camp
8,300m / 27,231ft

South Summit

South Col

Baruntse
7,162m / 23,497ft

Hillary Step

Lhotse
Face

Geneva Spur
7,950m / 26,083ft

The Balcony
8,300m / 27,231ft

Camp Two
(Green Tent)
7,400m / 24,278ft

Nuptse
7,861m / 25,791ft

Camp Four
7,950m / 26,080ft

Camp Three
7,000m / 22,966ft

Base Camp,
North Side

Changtse
7,543m / 24,747ft

North Col

North
Face

Southwest
Face

Camp Two
6,400m / 20,997ft

Western Cwm

China (Tibet)
Nepal

Camp One
5,950m / 19,521ft

Rongbuk Glacier

Lho La

Khumbu Icefall

Scale varies in this perspective.

**Everest and the
Landmarks of Learning**

Base Camp Nepal

Khumbu Glacier

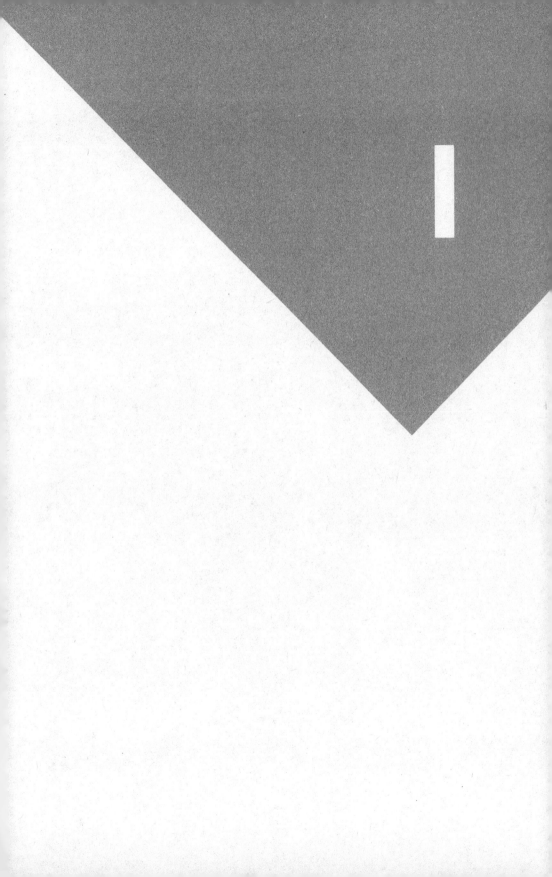

I

1.

MASQUERADE

2010: Mount Everest, Nepal

"*You are in the death zone. You are dying.*" I wiggled around, trying to create enough space to take a breath. My knit hat felt too tight on my head and I adjusted it, hoping to relieve the squeeze. Nothing changed. It was not my hat that was too tight; it was my skull. The pressure created a dull pain and discomfort that was a warning to my body.

The narrow walls of the two-person tent felt cramped and suffocating. My temporary shelter of yellow nylon was perched five miles above sea level on the exposed rocks of the South Col, the highest camp on the Nepal side of Mount Everest. The punishing wind whipped against the fabric, pushing the sides of the tent against my tired body. It was a warning of what might be ahead. It was a reminder of the immensity of my desire to reach the top of the highest place on Earth for the third time, without using supplemental oxygen for this attempt.* Doing it this way tests the human capacity to endure pain and challenges the rules of physiology, and so would, I hoped, answer the question of whether or not I was good enough. If I could answer that, maybe I could put down the weight of all the other questions I was carrying.

My headlamp beam illuminated my breath as I exhaled, and the wispy vapors saturated the small space, freezing and turning into a sparkling coat of ice on the inside of the tent walls. The sun had already descended below Nuptse, the mountain to the west of Everest, casting a dark shadow over the camp. The smell of musty nylon mixed with the sweet scent of black tea steeping in an open thermos in my hands. I looked straight into the darkness, my torso slouched forward with my elbows resting on my thighs.

Everything felt too crowded. I had shoved my legs inside my down suit, and the suit inside my sleeping bag, and my sleeping bag into the tiny space next to Dave Morton, my climbing partner. He was in his sleeping bag surrounded by everything we needed for the summit bid that night. Tshering Dorje Sherpa was in a tent next to us with another Tshering Sherpa whom he had hired to work with him that season.† They were both high-altitude workers and were the only other members of our team on the mountain.

Tshering Dorje and Dave had been with me two years before, on my first summit of Everest. Tshering Dorje had a raspy voice from the drying effects of the high-altitude air, and it made everything he said sound like a wise whisper. He was gentle and focused, a former monk who had left the monastery to make a living as a climbing guide. He married a strong-willed Sherpa woman and had two beautiful and equally strong-

---

* Throughout the book I will mention climbing "without oxygen," which actually means climbing without *supplemental* oxygen.

† Traditionally, Sherpas are named after the day of the week they are born on. Middle names are given based on gender and their last name is Sherpa. So 150,000 Sherpas have some combination of the same name. It is hard to keep straight but important.

willed daughters. I liked to think that we got along so well because he was used to being surrounded by women who were like me, even though he always reminded me that, like most women, I talked too much. His words, in contrast, were few, and always well considered.

After our first year climbing together, he cast a few of his well-chosen words my way. "You have good luck, Didi. Very lucky." He called me Didi, which means "big sister" in the Nepali language. His words made me feel like a valued member of a family I didn't know I had. I adored his perspective and ached to make it my own. But my luck had never been particularly noteworthy. And now, as I considered the task in front of me from the cold tent, I knew even the luck I did have wouldn't be enough.

We had been climbing that day for almost eleven hours before we reached the tent. I had watched the sun rise and now it was setting. The torturously slow pace ensured that I felt every moment, footstep, and uphill movement through my entire body, and my mind was weighted down with the unknown of the climb to come. Discomfort's persistent voice told me not to stay here for long. Otherwise, I might end up staying forever, just like the body left on the slope above us, frozen in place for fifteen years. He was a climber doing the same thing I came here to do, to climb without oxygen. A climber who fell victim to Mother Nature's power and the finality she promises us all.

Climbing to the highest point on Earth without supplemental oxygen was thought to be physiologically impossible until Reinhold Messner and Peter Habler did it in 1978. It took another ten years for a woman to do the same, and in the twenty-two years that followed, only three more women succeeded at the challenge, with one of them, an American woman named Francys Arsentiev, making it to the top but dying on the descent. Hundreds of climbers tried but failed for various reasons. Some failures were as mundane as losing motivation, others as gruesome as blackened fingers and toes falling off with frostbitten tissue. Some people died.

Nature conquers the desires of man in this way. At these altitudes, the lack of oxygen and the increase in pressure cause brain tissue to swell until the tiny blood vessels no longer have enough space to carry vital oxygen-rich blood to the body. The pressure increase will cause fluid to leak into the lungs, drowning them in death. High altitude is no place to live for long.

The successful climbs without oxygen proved that it was possible, but not for just anyone. Was it possible for me? I had wondered. Could I rise above being average, a place where I had resided most of my life? Average had allowed me to get here, but the intoxicating possibility that I could be more was pushing me forward and begging me to risk it all. If I could do this, I could do anything.

When I asked Dave to join me on this expedition, he said yes, simply and calmly. His lack of pause made me believe that he thought it was possible as well, so I began planning and dreaming about how we would make it happen as a tiny team of two. Dave had begun his career in the Himalayas twenty years earlier, and it showed in both the way he moved confidently and the community that knew him well. He was my mentor on my first trip to Everest a few years earlier, and I had forced him into a friendship with the persistence of a little sister. Quiet and patient, Dave was a good listener and quick to laugh. He would argue for days about the merit of a given Scrabble word and then just as easily concede that he was wrong. He had seen me grow over the years as I gained more experience in the big mountains. I was still learning the intricate ways of Everest, but his continued willingness to be my partner gave me a certain comfort. It was just us against nature.[*]

"I'm glad the wind calmed down after the Yellow Band." Dave looked at me as he spoke from his sleeping bag. No matter where you are, people talk about the weather when they don't know what else to say.

I took the deepest breath I could and choked my words out. "This is as high as I have ever been without oxygen. I can't believe I made it." Insecu-

---

[*] It would take me years to learn the secret that nature isn't your competitor but your teacher. And the teacher always wins.

rities flooded my mind. Dave was already tucked in, drinking tea, and organizing his camera gear for the final climb in a few hours, but I was so nervous that I couldn't hold still or do anything productive. My throat was so tight and full of emotion that I could barely breathe. I wanted to cry but I thought it would reveal my weakness. In my sleeping bag, I wrestled my way out of my underlayers, wet with sweat, and replaced them with the dry ones I had selected for the summit push. Under my down suit I wore a pair of insulated pants. Under those I wore my favorite pair of soft wool long underwear. And under all the other layers, I wore a pair of blue satin underwear I had stolen from my sister in high school. They were silky and feminine, and as a teenager I had hidden them away for when I had the confidence to wear them myself. I had worn them on each of my previous Everest summits. There was something rebellious about bringing something so delicate to such a harsh environment. On my first climb, I thought that if I died, at least I would die in pretty undies.

Each day of this expedition had been a seesaw of feeling that I was capable, strong, and able or that I was incompetent, weak, and a complete fraud. Both feelings only intensified as we got closer to the possibility of the summit, and now, after sixty days, they were my persistent partners, joining my every step.

"What do you think, Melis?" Dave asked gently, as was his way. I sucked in a deep breath and forced it out with a little whistle. Could I go any farther without oxygen? My head throbbed and my throat tightened. Lactic acid pulsed through my muscles, making them feel heavy and useless with fatigue. My heart pumped forcefully, and I imagined it pleading with my brain to just let me try.

I rubbed my hands together to warm them and then placed my palms over my eyes, darkening my world while scanning the backs of my eyelids for the answer. Why wasn't there someone I could call who could tell me what to do next? I heard my first climbing mentor and boss, Peter Whittaker, in my head: *Tag the top, everyone will celebrate and love you.* I heard voices from my childhood: *You're worthless. No one can love you.*

I thought about all the hard and impossible-seeming things I had done. I wasn't afraid of discomfort. The discomfort was more familiar to me than nearly anything else. I thought about my teen years, and how pain had seemed infinite and inescapable, but I had somehow made it through. I recalled cleaning hotel rooms and working at health clubs to save enough money to survive and escape to something better. I thought about all the times I had run away, and how it mostly had been trading in one form of discomfort for another. I knew how to escape, move on, and never look back. What was foreign to me was staying, living in the pain, and solving its puzzle. The physical discomfort of doing the hardest thing I had ever done was amplified in my mind by the discomfort of not knowing if I even deserved to be here trying.

I uncovered my eyes with another deep breath and looked at Dave. He had an oxygen mask on his lap, and he was adjusting the straps and checking the valves. The bottle that it would attach to sat beside him—a narrow cylinder about the height of a backpack. It weighed eight pounds and contained hours of a luscious and life-sustaining element. Inside that oxygen tank was the ability to climb faster, stay warmer, and think more clearly. Inside that tank, the summit was all but guaranteed.

But inside that tank, there was also failure. I wanted to show myself to the mountain and the world. I wanted to prove that I could survive at the highest point on Earth, just as I was. That all I needed was within me. That I was enough.

I exhaled and whispered my words to Dave. "I don't know."

A gust of wind crashed into the side of the tent violently, causing me to collapse further inward. I felt like a weak and wilted version of who I had hoped to be. I wasn't supposed to feel weak; I was supposed to feel powerful and capable of what was ahead. I closed my eyes again, wondering what I should do, afraid of either choice.

* * *

The journey that brought us to this cold night in the death zone on Everest had started nearly two months earlier with a simple hiking trail spanning thirty miles and cresting multiple mountain passes. It took ten days of hiking in the moody spring weather of early April for us to arrive at the 17,800-foot Everest Base Camp that would be our home for the months ahead. When we arrived at the massive but temporary village[*] of tents that composed Base Camp, we began resting our bodies and adjusting to the high-altitude air before slowly beginning to carry loads up higher on the mountain. The rhythm of our movement was all about repetition: Climb up, sleep at a new altitude, climb down, rest. Climb back up, higher this time, sleep, climb back down, rest again. Repeat.

It was amazing to watch ourselves adapt to the thinnest air on Earth in real time. A climb that could take five hours on the first rotation would be whittled down to a quick three-hour jaunt a month later. Progress was measurable.

Climbing Everest from the south side in Nepal involved rotating through a fixed set of numbered camps before reaching Camp Four at the South Col, at almost 26,000 feet. At each camp we would rest a few days and allow ourselves to adjust to the new altitude before heading back down to Base Camp. Up and down again and again, slowly higher each time.

The first obstacle above Base Camp on the way to Camp One was the Khumbu icefall, a constantly moving fortress of balancing ice blocks, most of them bigger than a suburban house. The high-altitude glaciers are frozen rivers, slowly flowing over the rocky cliffs they cling to. As the ice is beckoned by gravity, it will crack and shift in bursts, moving the blocks and occasionally starting a suffocating white avalanche, destroying everything in its path. We placed metal construction ladders over the deep cracks in the ice to make the route passable, but the constant movement of the glacier meant that the route was always changing.

---

[*] The camp, situated on the ever-melting ice at the foot of the Khumbu glacier, was put up and taken down each season. Over fifty teams would huddle in, with the entirety of the camp spanning almost a mile and filled with hundreds of personal tents and nearly just as many large dining tents. It was a circus of sorts, and we were the clowns.

Each change had to be learned until the puzzle of ice would slowly reveal a solvable sequence of ropes and ladders, ups and downs.

The headaches and shortness of breath lessened with each rotation. With time we could move quickly through, relearning the topography on each pass. Climbing quickly was the silent offering we made to the mountain gods, begging for safe passage.

The majority of the three hundred or so climbers on Everest that season were paying clients with various levels of experience, along with the guides who kept the novice climbers safe. For every international climber, there was at least one or two local workers, many of them Sherpa. They operated as the vital human infrastructure to make climbing this mountain possible by carrying loads, fixing ropes on the mountain, and guiding clients.* There was also a sprinkling of professional climbers, most pursuing new routes or oxygen-free ascents. They were the elite. They were exceptional. They were who I wanted to be. Most were well-known names, the royalty of international climbers: Gerlinde Kaltenbrunner, the Austrian woman who had climbed twelve of the fourteen highest peaks on Earth without oxygen; Ueli Steck, the Swiss speed climber who ran up vertical faces as though he were Spider-Man.

Dave and I existed somewhere between the guides and the elite climbers. Our friends were the guides; they spoke the language we knew well, and we would spend much of our time at Base Camp playing cards and hanging out with them. Occasionally, Gerlinde, Ueli, and the other elites invited us into their world, and I would do my best to act like I belonged. Ueli was focused on his plan to climb Nuptse, a steep and technical peak that shared a ridgeline with Everest's summit. He gave his

---

* Most of these workers were Sherpa, which is a tribe of people, and so much more than that. They are not just a job title. Capital S Sherpa are an ethnic group of people who migrated from Tibet. They make up the majority of local guides, load carriers, and route fixers on the big mountains in the Himalayas. But not all workers are Sherpa, so they are simply called high-altitude workers rather than the lowercase s "sherpa." (You might think these footnotes are annoying right now, but trust me, you will grow to love them. I put all my secrets here.)

opinion on the weather forecast with so few words, I imagined it must be how he did everything. Swiss. Efficient. Conserving energy. I was immediately envious in their presence. I wanted both to be seen by these climbers and to blend into the background before they noticed that I wasn't one of them. I hoped that proximity to their greatness could somehow make me great.

The season moved forward in the rhythm of our movement, slow but intentional. We survived each pass through the icefall. We set up our tents higher and higher on the mountain, at Camp Two and then at Camp Three. We swaddled our frozen fingers in warm down mittens for the early-morning climbs up the nearly vertical face of the Lhotse headwall, the steepest pitch of the climb that allowed us passage between Camps Two and Three and eventually onward to the South Col, in the death zone. Through good weather and bad, we kept pushing up, higher and closer to where we wanted to be.

We had waited as other teams had gone on their summit bids earlier that season, and had endured the anxious feeling that we were letting the only good weather pass. As we waited at Base Camp, metal wrenches banged on the aluminum exteriors of oxygen cylinders to announce that another team had touched the top of the earth. We connected our satellite internet each day to download a new weather forecast from a meteorologist who specialized in Himalayan forecasts. We agonized over the long-term outlook, drank hot tea, and hoped we weren't making a mistake by waiting. If everything worked out, our patience would be rewarded by a less crowded late-season opportunity to get to the summit.

The challenge was that we didn't just need a good-weather window; we needed a perfect one. Getting to the summit while using supplemental oxygen requires decent weather, but to safely summit without oxygen, everything had to come into alignment. Without the use of oxygen, we would be slower and need a longer window of calm skies to climb up and back down. With an average summit temperature of minus thirty degrees Fahrenheit, a light wind could blacken the tip of my nose and fingers with frostbite. Experience had taught me that the closer the calendar inched toward June, the warmer the days would be.

Like most of the decisions at high altitude, the wait was a tradeoff. With that June warmth would come moisture and wet afternoon snow that could decrease visibility and lead to new avalanche hazards. The formerly frozen ice on the lower flanks of Everest would begin to melt and become slushy, exposing cracks too large to cross and icy lakes that we could easily plunge into.

We ultimately timed our summit bid for May 24. I had summited on May 22 and May 23 in my two previous climbs, and it felt seren-dipitous to follow the sequence. We made the plan after most of the work was behind us. We had already made four rotations up and back down from various camps high on the mountain. We had descended to a village below Base Camp at 14,000 feet to breathe in extra oxygen and eat baked goods before our final ascent. We had moved methodi-cally uphill on our final pass through the Khumbu icefall, passing Camp One and heading straight to Camp Two, which was above 22,000 feet. We had rested a day there, eating cheese sandwiches and drinking lemon tea while waiting for the most current weather forecast to give us permission to continue. We climbed efficiently and together up the steep and glistening ice of the Lhotse face to a small perch at Camp Three.

After nearly sixty days of toil, we had made our way above Camp Three for the first time, committing to a summit attempt as we inched toward the death zone. We were headed to the South Col, Camp Four, and the small yellow nylon tent on the flat, football field–size outcrop-ping that was the highest camp on Everest, just one day of climbing away from the summit. The slope up to it was undulating but remained nearly vertical for over two thousand feet.

We didn't speak much as we climbed, conserving our energy for the unknown that was sprawled out ahead of us. I tried to visualize how Ueli moved, nearly floating uphill, and tried to merge that ease with my own clunky movements. I stood as straight as I could with each step, one leg bent in front of me and all my weight resting on the other leg, locked and straight. With my weight divided between a carefully placed crampon dug into the hard alpine ice and the rest of my weight hanging from the rope that was anchored to the mountain above me, I would pull up and step up, each movement heavy but precise. There was a thousand feet of air below my feet as they kicked into the icy steps on the firm, nearly vertical glacier. Each step would be accompanied by five long deep breaths in an attempt to slow my rapidly beating heart. The whole cycle—step, breathe, breathe, breathe, breathe, breathe, pull, and step again—took more than a minute to complete. Then I would swing the straight leg uphill past the bent leg and they would change positions. The movement had the robotic effect of a techno dance, far from floating and infinitely slower. With an oxygen tank I could have easily maintained a forward-flowing pace instead of this choppy series of rests. But movement was movement.

As the hours passed, I slowly made my way over the icy bulges above Camp Three. At this point, any climbers who were ascending toward their own summit bids had already strapped on their oxygen masks and moved past us. I resented their ease.

To climb Everest, we used ropes anchored to the mountain instead of a single rope attaching us to each other, which allowed us to move at different paces while staying anchored to the slope in case of a fall. As we moved closer to the South Col, I occasionally allowed my gaze to drift up and I would see Dave ahead of me, moving farther away each time. I tried to convince myself that everything was fine and at each pause for breath I would whisper to myself, "You've got this, you can do this." But my heart pounded heavily, trying to absorb what little oxygen was available. My body flooded with discomfort as nature pushed firmly against my desires.

By the time I climbed awkwardly over the sunshine-colored marble and quartzite stone of the Yellow Band, I was behind Dave by more than a few minutes. I pulled on the fixed ropes, heaving myself uphill against the ever-increasing gravity, finding it perplexing that the air began to feel so heavy as it quite literally thinned. How could such thin air provide such tremendous resistance? It seemed that oxygen had been replaced by gravity.

The day had been inching by at the same pace as my sloth-like movements, and now the afternoon sun was nipping at the edge of the Nuptse wall. The South Col was not close. I still had to climb the thousand-foot buttress of rock that makes up the Geneva Spur. I knew that as soon as the sun fell behind the wall the air temperature would drop below freezing, so I stopped and wrestled my way into my down suit, all while staying tethered to the ropes that were attached to the mountain. I was barely moving, and yet breathing as hard as a heavyweight boxer who somehow had made it to the tenth round. I zipped the suit and wrapped myself into the warmth and familiarity it provided. I looked up again. Dave was now out of sight. I guessed that he was already over the Spur. A lump of tension rose in my throat.

My eyes scanned the slope above me, looking for a place to rest, but tears quickly clouded my vision. The confidence I had started this expedition with had grown as thin as the air around me. My doubts began to thump in my ears in a contrasting rhythm to my heartbeat. I was alone because I could not keep up. I was alone because I was not strong enough to keep up. I could not do this. Why did I ever think I could? I had never been exceptional at anything, and only exceptional people could climb Everest without oxygen. I was not one of the elites. Who cared that I had easily gotten to the top twice before? Who cared that I trained all year? I was weak and slow and, now, alone.

I thought about everyone who knew I was making this attempt. I hadn't been afraid to tell people—I was going to be the first American woman to climb Everest without supplemental oxygen and survive the descent! The more I shared this audacious goal, the more I started to believe it could be true. I scoured the faces of those I told, trying to see whether they believed or doubted me.

I had already been lauded as not only an Everest summiteer, but a *woman* Everest summiteer—and yet there always seemed to be qualifications. My mother had shared a clipping from *Outside* magazine about my climb with the annual family Christmas letter, adding that I was no longer floundering and had found a path. The warm praise and the cold blade. *Floundering. Found a path.* I wanted to be irrefutably considered capable. I wanted to hush the whispers about how I only got to guide on Everest because the male bosses and clients thought I was cute. I wanted to forget the voice of the client I guided my first year on Rainier who refused to call me anything other than "Hotcakes," and the snickers from my peers that I only had a sponsorship because of my relationship with the head of the guide service—and the perception of what I might be doing in exchange for that. I wanted to silence it all, to prove that I wasn't here because of luck, beauty, or my perceived usefulness as a female. I wanted to belong. I wanted to be all the things the *Women's Health* article printed after my second summit said I was: a badass, an inspiration, a trailblazing high-altitude mountaineer. But as night absorbed the remaining daylight, as my pace slowed and my mind raced, all the things I wanted seemed further away than ever.

As I inched my way along the route toward the yellow tent with Dave waiting there for me, I knew I would have to decide whether I would risk it all and push forward toward the summit without oxygen. But now I also knew that I was not exceptional. I wasn't badass. I couldn't float up vertical slopes like Ueli Steck. You cannot wish a new truth into existence.

As I made the final, torturously slow climb into camp and my eyes lit upon the small yellow tent that had seemed out of reach all day, I let out the breath that had been trapped in the base of my lungs. Emotion rose in my throat as I watched the wind shake the tent. I remembered sitting on the couch in my parents' house as a teenager, GED in hand, getting ready to move out before I even turned eighteen because our relationship had become fractured beyond repair. I could see my father's eyes, curiously wondering what I would make of myself. I could hear my mother's words, adding weight to my already too heavy mind. *You are a liar. You are selfish. Nobody wants you around. No one trusts you.* And now, as I stood battered by the mountain, her words felt like the truth.

I pulled my mind back to the final steps in front of me and the sim-plicity of my movement as the last light of the day spotlighted the truth. No matter who I wanted to be, this is who I was. I was alone. I was too slow to keep up with Dave. I might be able to climb Everest, but I couldn't do it without the help of oxygen. I wasn't elite; I was barely average.*

I crested the Geneva Spur to see Tshering Dorje leaning on a rock outcropping, waiting patiently for me. He had been there for a while, I could tell. "Are you okay, Didi?" he asked in his signature raspy whisper.

We slowly covered the final traverse that brought us to our camp and the tiny tent shaking in the wind. He helped me get my pack off and undo my crampons. I did not want help. I wanted to do it by myself, and I felt the defiance of a toddler rise as I shrugged him away. But I didn't have the strength to refuse. Every ounce of strength I had was being used to keep me from collapsing.

* * *

Now the oxygen mask sat like a threat in Dave's lap. He held still, draped in a relaxed comfort that felt foreign to the turmoil inside me. He was always so calm, and sitting here in the death zone he was no different. It was time to decide. Was I enough? Could I do this? Should I even still try?

"I feel like we need to be able to get to the summit in twelve hours," he said. "It took us almost that long to get here today, and it was only two thousand feet. Tonight will be three thousand feet and much harder. Do you think you could move any faster?"

---

* I know this may seem like a ridiculous thing to say. You might be thinking that average people don't summit Everest multiple times. But they do. It is how I have made my living, being an average person helping other average people do hard things. It is my favorite thing about the mountains: You don't have to be anything special to climb them. You just have to be willing to suffer and then quickly forget how hard it all is so you do it again.

"I can't go faster," I said in the near whisper of a single exhale, avoiding eye contact with him.

He didn't look at me either but continued to fiddle with the oxygen mask for a few eternal seconds until he finally set it on my lap. "It's up to you."

Dave had his own oxygen mask already firmly sealed on his face, and as I looked at this spare mask meant for an emergency, I could not tell if I wanted it to be up to me. I could not tell if I felt devastated or relieved. I let my fingers wander over the edge of the rubber mask, barely touching it but fully aware of its weight. I took another deep breath and exhaled, letting this last moment of my dying dream sit in the overcrowded space.

I picked up the mask as Dave slid the oxygen tank next to me and turned the regulator on, allowing the slow hiss of oxygen to begin to escape. I wanted to escape, too. Instead, I slipped the mask over my head and nestled it on my nose, feeling the seal suction itself to my cheeks and chin. I took a breath.

With each breath, my headache slipped away and my fingers and toes warmed up. The low level of nausea that marked my time above Camp Two gave way to the first hunger I had truly felt in over a month. I despised how good this failure felt in my body. Dave quietly prepared his remaining things, and we shared some ramen noodles before closing our eyes for a few hours. He did not talk about it anymore. He just moved on to our new plan to get to the summit together, both with oxygen. I wished I could just move on, too, but my mind was already navigating the justifications that I would have to make when we got down. Soon everyone would know what I had known all along—that I was not exceptional.

We awoke after midnight and climbed out of the tent an hour later, fully dressed and both wearing our oxygen masks and carrying two tanks in our backpacks. We looked like overdressed scuba divers and moved around clunkily, as though we had flippers instead of crampons. I tucked a hot water bottle into the chest of my down suit and double-checked that I had spare headlamp batteries. The Tsherings crawled out of their tent and together the four of us climbed, swiftly and steadily. I felt strong and capable, protected now by the hissing flow of oxygen, with the mask obscuring my face. But I also felt hollow. My emotions waged a war inside me. We passed a few other teams as we ascended the steep rock and ice of the Triangular Face toward the Balcony and our first real break for a quick sip of water and an attempt at swallowing a frozen Snickers bar. Our metal crampons scraped over the rocks with spine-cooling screeches as we made our way up the mountain. The snow supported us, crunching under our crampons as we attached ourselves to the fixed ropes and moved uphill in unison. We arrived at the Balcony before the sun, silently agreeing to just keep moving for warmth. I wondered how different this would be if I didn't have the mask on. I was curious about how cold I would feel and if I would be able to keep moving. The Southeast Ridge rose above us steeply and we continued our movement, dancers on a rope, mimicking one another's steps.

The sun was rising over the Tibetan plateau, illuminating the four-sided pyramid of Makalu, the fifth-highest peak in the world, just thirty miles south of Everest. We dipped into the notch at the south summit and traversed easily to the Hillary Step. We climbed over it and balanced precariously on the sloping shale rocks that lead to the summit ridge.

It was still early, but the sun was well above the horizon as we took the final steps onto the summit, just the four of us. It had felt only as strenuous as a hard summit day on Rainier, and I resented the oxygen for depriving me of the challenge I so desperately wanted.

The mountain had exposed me. There was no spinning it or hiding it now. All the discomforts I had endured in my life still weren't enough to make me capable of getting through this. I wanted to be seen, to shed all the lies and layers and shadows and belong, irrefutably. The failure felt heavy. I exhaled as the weight of my entire life and all the choices that had brought me to this point settled into the front of my mind.

2.

FENCES

1988: Southern Colorado

"Get out of my fucking face!" My mother's words hit me like a punch. I fought back tears as I fled to my room, shutting the door and slumping to the ground, hugging my five-year-old knees close to my chest. The skin on my face was hot. What had I done? What broken rule had woken her rage today? Last week I had hidden under my bed some Rice-a-Roni noodles that I had spat into a napkin at dinner. Maybe she found them? Then I remembered: I had gone to work with my dad at a construction site the day before, and the owners of the house he was working on had told her how well-behaved I was. I shivered, wondering if that could be it. Being bad and breaking rules was worthy of punishment, but being praised and loved was worthy of hate.

My mother was a creature of intense habit. Every day she would wake up in the dark early-morning hours and have her first cigarette of the day as soon as she left bed. It seemed to me that she would start her day angry because she just wanted to sleep but her pain meant that she never could. Her pain had no consistently identifiable origin, but it had personality. Sometimes it was her back that hurt and other times it was a pinched nerve in her arm. Sometimes it just seemed to come from the resentment of being stuck in a small trailer with small children. But wherever the pain came from, it inevitably turned to anger.

She collected her weed from a dark brown rolltop stash box, grabbed her pipe, book, and pain pills, and settled herself into the graying old chair that leaned to the right from years of holding her weight. Her lighter flicked and ignited a crackle, producing the pungent, sticky smell that coated the house, turning musty and stale over time. The act of being stoned was meant to numb her from the pain, but it seemed to me that it only sensitized her to the discomfort, magnifying it until it burst into flames. The pain robbed her of any tolerance for daily life, morphing her into a raging bear with big sharp teeth, an animal you aren't meant to see up close.

Did you know some mother bears eat their own cubs? Mammalian mothers are required to nurse their young immediately after they are born, and if the mother bear cannot find enough food for herself or deems the cub unfit to survive, she will kill and eat it. In my five-year-old mind, my mother morphed into that type of mother bear nearly every day, assessing her cubs for their fitness to survive and threatening to eat them if they couldn't prove their worth. After all, she didn't even want cubs. I knew my origin story to be one of burden. I remember her saying it all the time—"I never wanted kids"—like it wasn't personal, but each repetition only pressed on the raw abrasion on my heart.

That she didn't want *me* in particular was clear in the way I was punished for things that went unremarked on when my sister, Stephanie, was the culprit. Although we came from the same family and she was barely a year older than me, it seemed to me that we were different animals altogether. She was pale-skinned, brown-haired, and quick to bruise with the slightest bump. I was tan and blond, with scars covering the tough skin of my legs. She was shy, obedient, and a budding perfectionist. I was extroverted, rebellious, and messy.

But we balanced each other. Close in age, we formed an unspoken alliance. We shared our toys and our space and our secrets. We marveled at how different we were, unsure of who had the advantage in each situation life presented us. Still, I was envious of her ease within our family. She knew something that I had yet to discover, and this little revelation and her ability to abide by it made all the difference in our lives: She knew how to avoid the roaring wrath of the bear. I often watched, mystified, at how she managed to sidestep the fury so gracefully. I admired it, but not enough to change.

Every rebuke told me I was unworthy to live in this den. In the car, I sat behind my father and diagonal from my mother. If my sister and I were playing too loudly, it was me who was in the path of that giant, angry bear paw. I might have appeared to be the misfit little bear cub, but as the days sped by, I was starting to think I wasn't even a bear at all. With each punishment I took, and each my sister avoided, it became clearer that I didn't understand how bears lived and so I could never become one.

* * *

Our property was nestled inside the arid, high desert just south of the San Juan Mountains. At the northeast corner of the land sat our trailer, long and skinny with tiny bedrooms; thin brown panels for walls; and a cream-colored linoleum kitchen floor tinged yellow from my mother's cigarette smoke. The trailer was situated far away from the road and any neighbors, and our lives were hidden inside.

The trailer was meant to be a temporary home. My dad was going to build us a beautiful cabin with an upstairs and a big bedroom for everyone. I dreamed about that cabin until it became clear that it would never be built. Instead, we enclosed the temporary foundation around the trailer and planted tulips and a yard of soft green grass. It was the only home we knew in Colorado. We would live there until I turned twelve and everything changed.

My dad was tall and sturdy, with long dark brown hair pulled into a ponytail that snaked down his back. His face was obscured by a beard that reached the middle of his chest. If you didn't look closely, he could appear like a grizzly—fierce and protective. But if you saw his dark brown eyes, surrounded by soft skin that was quick to wrinkle when he laughed, you would know that this bear was gentle. He affectionately referred to me as Turtle, a nickname he had given me when I was a toddler tucked inside his adult-size T-shirts.

My dad had a deep sense of commitment, to my mom and to us girls. He had met my mother in 1978 when he was working in Colorado. He worked construction all summer, and when the sites shut down in the winter, he went into the mountains to take shifts as a ski patroller. He was easygoing and hardworking and loved to spend his days outside. One of his most defining personality traits was his antiestablishment, antigovernment sentiment, which manifested in a "peace, love, and ganja for all" vibe. He didn't make much money, but we had what we needed, and I knew he would rather pound nails for pennies than collect a check from the authority he disdained.

It was on one of those days pounding nails and soaking in the southern Colorado sun that the accident happened. After surgery and a long hospital stay, he came home to weeks spent in bed, recovering from a terrible back injury. Uncertainty and sadness consumed the trailer. He brought the only income to our family, and after the accident there was none. We had no insurance. We survived on canned food donations from a church we didn't go to, sustained by visits from fellow hippie friends who lived in their vans and understood what it meant to stretch a penny. My mother was tasked with holding our entire family together, caring for us kids and now for him, too, while trying to solve the miserable puzzle of our survival.

The weight of this challenge changed something in my father. He went from being bedridden to slowly using a cane, and when he had learned to walk again, he put on an ironed white shirt and brand-new Wrangler jeans and went to town to get a desk job.

His new office was in the center of the small town, just down the street from my elementary school, amid rows of drab houses and apartments with pink and yellowing adobe exteriors. These were the government HUD houses that my dad now managed, many of which were inhabited by members of the Southern Ute tribe. My dad's job intertwined our family life with the tribe's. Sometimes the relationship could be adversarial, but mostly they folded us into their sacred rituals and ignored that it was we, the white people, who were forcing them to live there. My first-grade teacher, Ms. Pinnacuse, was Southern Ute, and she taught me the names of colors in her language. She wore beautiful turquoise rings on the hands with which she wrote me letters, always starting with "Máykh, Missy Girl," then continuing to blend English and Ute words together, trying to help me learn. The tribe's medicine man came to our school and bestowed us with parables explaining why the sun rose and why you should never trust a fox.

My parents were young and had limited resources to nurture a young family. They were different people who had wanted different things in life, but they made what they could of it, living in that silver trailer surrounded by a tall fence on the edge of the Southern Ute Indian Reservation. When they felt a reprieve from the stresses of raising two kids with limited resources, they would lean into family life and share some ease with us. We drove into the mountains on the occasional weekend and lounged by the riverside, everyone content in the vast space and open mountain air. We would save enough money to rent two movies, and we would watch them together as a family. My parents were fully committed to each other, and when things were good, they put in the effort to smooth out the roughest edges of our lives. My mother took on the role of housewife and mom, doing her best to forget about any dreams she may have had for herself. She kept the house, no matter how imperfect it was, in perfect order.

She strived to keep me, an unruly and wild child, in the same sort of order. Her attempts to contain me came mostly in the form of punishments. I was grounded to my room for not finishing my chores. I had to

sit on a chair in the hallway for the entire weekend because I lied about returning a library book. My bedroom door had a little hook-and-eye lock on the outside to keep me caged within if they needed to leave the house and wanted to ensure that I wouldn't sneak candy from the cupboard or rifle through things that were not mine. One day when my mother's pain was particularly bad, she made my sister and me pack every belonging in our rooms into paper grocery bags and cardboard boxes as though we were moving out. But once she had carried all our toys and clothes and blankets to the shed and locked them in, she locked us in our empty rooms. It was meant to teach us some sort of lesson, but it felt like prison, like she wanted to both control me and ignore me. The conflict between these two poles made me feel uncertain where I belonged. Was I even loved? Or was I just tolerated? All I knew was that I didn't want to be controlled or ignored. The tighter the container she put around me, the harder I would fight my way out of it.

* * *

On one of the first days of kindergarten, I returned from a recess of swings and monkey bars to a classroom full of police. Seeing them made my heart race. My parents had instilled in us a deep distrust of police, explaining that they were just extensions of "the man." What had I done wrong now? Were they here to take me away? On the chalkboard at the front of the room hung a new black poster with bright red letters: D-A-R-E.

Mrs. Stroud introduced the officers, telling us that D.A.R.E. stood for Drug Abuse Resistance Education, and that the police would be coming to our classroom sometimes to teach us about bad things that we should watch out for.* The first officer had a chest twice the size of

---

* My dad would later say he was a veteran, fighting the War on Drugs, and he had the scars to prove it.

any human I had seen before. He asked us if we knew about the difference between right and wrong, between good and bad. Then he showed us pictures. White powder. Needles. Little rocks that looked like sparkly crystals. These were drugs, he explained, and they were always wrong, always bad. When he put up the picture of green leafy plants, I realized what I had known, on some level, all along: My mother's weed was wrong. It was bad.

I knew it must be a secret because of how she hid the pipe and the stash box away. When someone pulled unexpectedly up the driveway, she shoved the box hurriedly out of sight. Now I knew why: She was breaking the law. She was wrong. All along I had been the one getting in trouble but now I knew: *She* was the bad one. She was breaking the law, and it was okay for me to be mad at her. Even at this tender age, I knew that I was supposed to love my parents and trust them. But I didn't feel that, especially because I was always in trouble. Seeing the plants on the screen, I felt so good to find out that she, too, was in trouble. It wasn't just me. She couldn't hold her righteousness over me anymore. I savored this knowledge and stored it in a special place. I turned it over and over in my mind, feeling the weight of its power.

After the D.A.R.E presentation, Mrs. Stroud told us to draw a picture of our family. I sat at the round table, on the chair that was too tall for my feet to reach the floor. My wispy blond pigtails jutted out from the sides of my head, and my little fingers grasped the crayons with a fist. I daydreamed, as usual, as I formed the stick figures that represented my parents and sister. I drew a jagged and messy beard on the tallest stick figure to show that it was my father. I drew my sister with pigtails of her own. I drew the round and rigid figure of my mother. And I drew the dog, Mel, even though he was more like a stray dog than a member of the family. Mel was short for Milagro, or "miracle" in Spanish, but he was only ever called Mel, and I would jump when his name was called, unsure if it was a call for me or him. Our family had rescued him from his life as a stray dog. I was curious to watch the love and care my mother gave him even though she didn't have to. She fed him and brushed him and built a fence to keep him safe, though he simply jumped over it every night and ran off into the wilderness.

I envied his freedom. As I drew the stick figure family, I placed him at a distance from the people. I wanted that same distance. I wanted to jump my fence made of rules and boundaries I didn't understand and run off on great adventures. I wanted to be free. I wanted to form tangled little mats of hair that told the tale of the wild animal I was, instead of the neat pigtails that I was made to wear each day.

As I colored the blue eyes on my sister's figure, I began to turn my fantasy of running away into a plan. I would need my sister's help. Since she would be able to drive before I could, I decided that she would get a red convertible on her sixteenth birthday. The car would be fancy and fast, the opposite of our old broken-down two-door Subaru and my dad's clunky red work truck that almost never started. Together we would escape the imprisonment and build a life where breaking the rules didn't mean you were locked in your room all day and fed only plain bread and water so you would know what prison was like. A life where we wouldn't wake up each day to a smoky haze and a nervous curiosity as to whether the bear would be sedated or waiting to fight.

I dreamed about the day my sister would get the convertible. My life of captivity would end and my life of adventure would begin. We would climb into the car, roll the top down, and speed into town. We would pull up to the yellowing brick building with all the police cars parked out front. We would tell them about the drugs and my mother would evaporate into the place where people who broke the law went. She would no longer be there to keep me captive. I would jump the fence just like Mel had been doing for years, but instead of returning to the little doghouse, I would burn down the house and there would be no returning.

3.

REVELATIONS

1993: Southern Colorado

The school bus stopped and we climbed down the steps and out onto the pavement of the county road. The driver waved us across, and before my feet even touched the dirt, I saw Bobbi waving excitedly at Stephanie and me. "What's Bobbi doing down here?" Steph asked me, both curious and confused. My sister was a fifth-grader now and in middle school. I was still in elementary school and almost ten years old. We usually walked home from the bus stop alone each day, savoring our last moments of independence before returning to the uncertainty of my mother's moods. But today, Bobbi met us. Something was up.

"Youns are going to come to my house. Your folks will grab youns later." Bobbi spoke with an accent that sounded like a mix of Irish and Deep South. She was in her sixties and had the quintessential grandmother look: a swoop of silver-white hair wrapped in a neat French twist. She was less than five feet tall, with the warped and weathered hands of a woman who got things done. Somehow, she had tricked my suspicious mother into being friends, a task at which I had seen nearly no one succeed. Bobbi often invited my sister and me over to help her water her rows and rows of rosebushes or feed her pond ducks. It was always a welcome time away from our home. But now Bobbi was whisking us to her house unplanned after school. I thought this could only be something very good or something truly terrible.

Bobbi fed us oatmeal cookies and milk, and we tossed cracked corn to the ducks as we waited, shuffling our feet anxiously in the dusty driveway near the duck pond. Bobbi seemed nervous, not ever letting her eyes catch mine, and this in turn made me nervous.

My parents' old car pulled into the driveway in the late-afternoon light, and they climbed out. Bobbi met them on the porch while Steph and I gathered our things. Adult whispers were exchanged, along with quick hugs as we greeted our parents. My dad spoke slowly and hushed, "Let's go, girls. Time to get you home." It sounded perfectly normal, but I knew it wasn't.

"Where were you?" I asked as soon as we climbed into the car.

"We need to talk to you girls," my dad responded in his deep hushed tone as our car bumped over the potholes and washboards on the short mile of hard-packed dirt road that led from Bobbi's house back to ours. That wasn't good. Talks were never good. Talks meant we were in trouble—that we would be given the chance to disclose what we had done wrong before they did, and we would sit and squirm, wondering what we should admit to. Dread filled my little body on the short five-minute drive to our house. "Go put your backpacks away and meet us in the living room." My mom spoke with a steady voice, which was worse than yelling. It was the seismic calm before the volcano erupted.

When we were settled, my dad sat down in his faded recliner. My mom sat in her own chair, with the little dark brown octagonal table separating them. It was spring and the sun hadn't set yet, and the golden glow of early evening coated the room. My dad stroked his long beard with his hand, as he was apt to do when he was nervous. "We need to tell you girls something," he began as Steph fidgeted on the couch and I picked at a little thread on the cushion that was beginning to unravel. So much was beginning to unravel now—I could feel it coming. I hugged my knees to my chest and switched to picking at the frayed ends of my jeans. "Today, your mom and I were arrested for growing pot plants. Marijuana. Someone called the cops, and they came and found some plants we had, and we were arrested." He paused. My sister began to cry. "It's okay, it's going to be okay. We broke the law, and listen, we disagree with the law. Pot isn't harmful—it's just a plant—but still, it isn't allowed, and we got caught, so now we have to face the punishment."

Tears continued to pour down Stephanie's face. Meanwhile, I had to suppress the giddy feeling forming deep in my belly. For once, I wasn't the one in trouble—it was *them*. For the first time in my life, I had the upper hand. They were getting grounded, not me. They were losing privileges, not me. I pulled the hood of my sweatshirt closely around my neck and tried to look sad.

"I will have to live in a house run by the state for a little while," my dad continued. "They are letting me go to work, and I will be able to see you guys a few times, but that is it."

The potential joy I felt started to drain. He was going away. No—he was my safe harbor. I broke his monologue with urgency. "What about Mom?"

She glared at me as she lit another cigarette. "I am going to be taking care of you girls. Just like always. I have to do community service, but I don't know what that is yet." She blew white smoke toward the ceiling and rocked rigidly in her armchair.

No, no, no, I thought. This couldn't be happening. I was supposed to start baseball that spring. My dad was supposed to teach me. He was supposed to be there daily to ensure she didn't go off the deep end and lock us in our rooms again. What would happen now? This wasn't good at all.

"We understand this is hard," my dad continued. "And we will spend some time together as a family this weekend. We want to give you girls the chance to ask any questions. Anything at all. We will answer." I looked at them both, wondering if a moment like this would ever come again. One where I wasn't the bad one in the family. One where I was told I could ask anything. I had questions—oh yes, I had questions.

"Is the Easter Bunny real?" My words came out in a rush. I was pretty sure I had seen my dad hiding eggs that year.

"No, the Easter Bunny isn't real." He answered calmly, looking me directly in the eyes.

I continued with my new and surely short-lived power: "What about Santa?"

"No, Melissa. Santa isn't real either." He exchanged a glance with my mom. My world narrowed a bit as my parents faced us, and the big truth of what was happening coupled with the childish truths I was seeking. They had been arrested, almost losing everything and absolutely changing our lives forever. And here was their youngest daughter, nine years old, and she was worried about Santa. Santa wasn't real, but this was.

My dad went away for some amount of time, indeterminable to my child brain. My mom started working at the battered women's shelter for her community service, and when she finished her obligation, she applied for an administrative job in the office there and was hired. She seemed to enjoy the job. I wonder now if it was, in part, due to being around women who were in such dire circumstances, making her feel better about her own life.

For a moment in time, a sweet and short moment, I thought the weed was gone. My mom didn't rush away to get high after every meal. She talked to us more, and her tone softened.* When my dad was released, they even took us to see the circus. Suddenly, my life was the one I had wished it to be, with two parents, no drugs, and the feeling of a place to belong where I was wanted.

It didn't last long. One day, through the closed bedroom door of the trailer, I smelled the familiar skunky smell seeping out, followed by the sound of her cough. I felt devastated. We had made it to a better place,

---

* I later learned that she never quit smoking weed, so that wasn't the reason for her change in tolerance and tone, though, I was sure that was why when I was a kid.

a good place, but now she had chosen weed over us. The seismic shift of this chain of events created a divide between us that became a piercing mountain range, rising jagged and unclimbable, creating a clear line of before and after. I would forever live in the after, no matter how hard I tried to climb back to the before.

* * *

I looked up, my hands still submerged in the lukewarm, soapy water of the dark brown dish bucket. There was a deep October darkness outside, and the only thing I could see in the window was my own reflection. I held my hands still, letting the smell of the fluffy white Dawn dish bubbles waft up as I looked into my own dark brown eyes.

My now eleven-year-old face was thin as my body struggled to grow into the woman I was becoming. I heard the muted coughs of my mother behind her closed bedroom door.

Who was going to notice that I was sad, I wondered? Who was going to pay attention to me? I had begun to dream of one day living in New York City or L.A. and far from the mountains I was raised in. It felt like no one could see the adult I was trying to become. I was unnoticed unless I did something wrong. Then I would be closely examined. Otherwise, it was just me and the infinite darkness of the night in front of me. The longer I looked into my own eyes, the more the edges of my vision became blurred by the threat of hot tears wanting to escape. I held them in, promising that if something was going to escape, it was going to be me.

The door burst open, startling me. "You aren't done with the dishes yet?" she snarled. "Go feed Mel and finish this!" I piled the leftover food onto a plate to deliver to the dog and slipped my feet into my dad's oversize Sorel snow boots without saying anything. When I got out to Mel's fence, I set down the dish and looked up at the late-fall sky. The air was cold and crisp, revealing the stars in perfect clarity. I breathed in the cold air and shivered in my plain white Hanes T-shirt. I wanted to live among the stars. I wanted to be free.

But something had changed, something my mom didn't know about. After years dreaming of escape, I finally knew just the way to get what I wanted.

That week at school, an office aide had shuffled into the classroom and handed a pink note to the geography teacher, Ms. Rose. I watched as she read the note and felt the flutter of anticipation so deep in my belly, it felt like it was shooting into my hips. "Melissa?" She motioned for me to come to the front of the class, and I exhaled, giddy and expectant. She handed me the small note and instructed me to take my things. I opened the pink paper and read, "Officer Jones needs to see you in the library." I grabbed my backpack and fled, taking deep breaths to calm my excitement. It had been almost two months of meeting with him, but it still felt special and wonderful. I wondered if this was what love felt like—irresistible and all-consuming.

He had dark black hair, a sturdy square build, and light brown skin. He wore a police uniform—black pants, short-sleeved black shirt, belt with a radio and a gun. He had a gold badge on his right chest pocket and a crooked scar that led from his upper lip to his nose. He was only twenty-six. He was so young that he seemed more like us kids than any of the adults we were used to being taught by.

The first day he came to our school and introduced himself, he said we could ask anything we wanted. Someone asked if he had ever killed anyone. He said that he had—a man who was growing pot farms and hiding from the law, he said. The police were told where the man was and when they went to arrest him, he came running at the officers with a knife, and Officer Jones had to shoot him.

I went home from school that day and told my parents the story. I wondered if it would scare them into giving up the pipe and the weed and all the attention it had stolen from me.

"I had a friend who was killed by the cops for growing weed," my dad said with a frown, his eyes creased all the way to his ears in distress. "The cops are pigs." I listened, trying to decide whose side I was on. But I already knew.

I started to wonder if Officer Jones could save me from the bear den that I didn't belong in. I hadn't yet felt the big emotions of something more than a crush. I hadn't yet entered the melancholic days of being a teenage girl. But I was starting to feel something different, and it electrified my desire to escape.

After the first weeks of D.A.R.E. that year, I could tell that Officer Jones was watching me. On my way to the playground one afternoon, he stopped me as I reached the door, asking if I would come sit at the picnic table outside and talk with him. I felt electricity pulse through my body. I was special. I was seen. He sat on top of the table, and I did the same, sitting next to him. I crisscrossed my legs and slumped forward, biting my cheek, waiting to hear his words. "I noticed you last week. I saw you looking at me like you have something you want to share. Your eyes look like they have pain in them."

He spoke softly and directly. I froze, unsure of what to say. My heartbeat felt faster than it ever had, and my skin felt hot. No one had ever asked me about my pain before. No one had ever said that my eyes had anything in them. And now here he was, just six inches away from me, telling me that he had noticed me.

"Well, I don't know. I mean. I sometimes . . . I just. I, um. You know that guy you killed? I told my parents about it. They do drugs too. I mean, they smoke pot. Not anything else. My mom does. My dad doesn't anymore, not since they got arrested for growing weed a few years ago. But my mom still does. And when I told them about your story, they told me about a friend of theirs that was killed by the cops too." My words tumbled out of my mouth quickly and in one breath. I sat still and inhaled, wondering what he would do. He reached over, touching my skinny child's knee with his adult hand. The weight of it felt heavy and warm on my leg as he spoke, still looking into my eyes.

"I am so sorry. Can I see you next week and we can talk some more?" I nodded, unsure of what I was agreeing to. He removed his hand and stood. I stood too, quickly mimicking his movements. "Can I give you a hug?" he whispered while reaching out for my shoulders and pulling me toward him, and with that embrace he began taking something I didn't even know I had.*

Our standard meeting place became the quiet corner of the library. The table was round, and it was hidden and dimly lit, tucked in the corner of an unused space. We would sit and talk, sometimes about me and sometimes about him. I learned that he had six kids. He had been married four times and was in the midst of getting another divorce.† He asked me questions about my life, and he listened. He sat for the whole story, no matter how long it was. He smiled and leaned in toward me, closer at each meeting, eventually touching me with his hands. He told me that I was special, and I was beautiful. I was going to be amazing as I grew up. He wanted me to be part of his life. He wanted me to be happy. He would rescue me from my pain, he said. I could come live with him, he said. He loved me, he said. And he would tell me stories about how we could leave Colorado and move to Texas. He would take me from my parents so that we could be together.

Being with Officer Jones became all I wanted. And each time he asked me to meet, I knew I was getting closer to that reality. On the day I got the pink note from Ms. Rose, I made my way down the hall to find him seated at the round table in the corner, like always. He stood as I approached and reached out, pulling my skinny preteen shoulders close to his body. I smelled his cologne and aftershave and hoped the smell would stick to me so I could enjoy it later. "How are you doing? I missed you this weekend." His words were whisper-like and gentle as he surveyed me. His eyes wandered from mine, down my body to my knee, where his hand had come to rest on my slightly dirty Kmart jeans.

---

* I often wonder how many young girls get crushes on their teachers or their parents' friends or some other unknowing adult in power and that adult doesn't act inappropriately. I wonder what would have happened if my first crush had been on one of those adults instead.

† In any other reality this would have seemed insane to me. But not in the reality I was in.

"The weekend was . . . like, it was fine," I said, being sure to convey sadness and need with my eyes by tilting my chin down and looking up, doe-like, at him. "I gave them the letter. They don't care. Or, whatever. They don't care about *me,* I mean." I pushed my words out nervously and slowly, wanting time to slow, wanting his approval.

I had already told him how I felt like my parents cared more about the drugs than they ever did about me. I filled in the details of my days with them and the lack of control I felt living with my mother and her unpredictability. And he listened. He offered me different ways of thinking about my life at home—ones that included being free from my parents. I had always thought the only way I would get out was to flee, but he told me that wasn't necessary. *They* could go away. Or, more accurately, they could be taken away. They were breaking the law. I could come and live with him. I could be free. With each morsel of attention he gave me, I only craved more.

When I told him I was sad, he would hold me close. So, I leaned all the way into my sadness and expanded it beyond its reality. When he had told me the previous week to write my parents a letter telling them I wanted them to stop smoking pot, I did it. I feared their wrath at my expectation that I, the kid, could tell them, the adults, what to do. But I did it for Officer Jones. And he rewarded me with more affection and attention. I was eleven. He was twenty-six. I was a sixth-grade student and he was a police officer and my teacher. And I loved him, never questioning if that was right or not. Never wondering why he was flooding me with attention and what he might want in exchange. It felt good to be wanted and be seen, so I committed to keeping his gaze on me, no matter what. I wasn't capable then of knowing what "no matter what" would truly mean.

Now he turned serious, almost grave. "It's time," he said. He spoke clearly and closely in a near whisper. "I have done everything I can here. You need to talk to the county sheriff." My parents were going away for a work trip to Denver in the months ahead, and all I had to do was tell the sheriff about how terrible my life was with them and I would be free. He told me that the Sheriff's Department would search the house and find the drugs; when my parents returned, they would get arrested and I wouldn't have to face them at all. "This is in the hands of the sheriff now; you will be safe. I will protect you," he promised with an embrace that felt both suffocatingly tight and like I was falling through space, held by nothing at all.

He promised to replace what I had known with something better. The idea seemed both unimaginable and inevitable. I started to meet him outside of school. I abandoned the child I had been, trying on what it felt like to be a woman. He pulled me abruptly out of my childhood and plunged me directly into his adult life. There was no way to uncross the line once it had been crossed.

* * *

In January my parents left town for their trip. My sister and I stayed with a family friend, only returning to our silver trailer once, to feed the cats. On Sunday I sat on Stephanie's bedroom floor and explained that I was telling the police on our mom and dad. "I don't believe you," she said as she reorganized her binders for school the next week. She looked up at me with disgust on her face. Her tone suggested that she maybe did believe me. She was in eighth grade, on the precipice of high school, and as I had gotten closer with Officer Jones, I had become more distant from her. She looked at me with suspicion, as though she knew I was up to no good. But I didn't feel I had the words to tell her everything. I shrugged and leaned against her wall, but I didn't try to convince her further. She would find out the truth soon enough.

I spent that night in my bed, wondering if I would ever sleep there again. I tried to memorize the look, and the feel, of my space. Everything was going to change, and it was because of me.

On Monday the sheriff came to school and took me out of class to wring all the details they could get from my young brain. He sat me at the small table inside the school counselor's office. "We need you to tell us everything you can, and don't leave out any details, okay, honey?" His voice conveyed the deep authority of a man in uniform. What had I seen? Were there plants? Were there pipes? What about a bong—did I know what that was? I told them everything I could, wondering if it was either not enough or far too much.

On Wednesday, while I was in school, the police came to the trailer with their search warrant and destroyed the house, looking for the drugs. A few hours after that, my sister went to feed the cats after school. I stayed at the house in town, afraid to return to the trailer, and I was curled in a chair reading when she burst back into the house where we were staying, having discovered our trailer searched and overturned recklessly. Her face was red and blotchy, as it often got when she was upset. She glared at me, saying nothing. My heart beat faster and my throat tightened as I realized that there was no going back. I was terrified and excited all at once, but mostly I was scared as I sat in silence near her. When my parents made their nightly check-in call from Denver, my sister spoke to them first. I lay on a bed in the room by the kitchen, not wanting to hear what she was saying. I knew what was happening. Change was coming. Change was here. My sister called my name, handing me the phone, and gazed at me with disgust. I wondered if the search warrant had said, "Melissa told on you." I wondered if Stephanie had told them it was my fault. I wondered if it was going to be my mom or my dad on the other end of the phone and I wondered what they knew.

"Hey, Turtle." It was my dad. The sweet nickname he called me my whole life. "I love you. We will be home Friday." That was it. I choked back the tears that were rising in my throat. I didn't know if he knew it was me. I wondered if he did know and chose to love me anyway. I hung up the phone and went back to the bed, crawling under the covers and hiding my head in the pillow. My sister came in and got into her side of the bed. She didn't say anything at all, but she looked like someone who had just been mugged. And she had been. I had just taken her security and left her with chaos. I hadn't considered what would happen next. I had only imagined that I would somehow be living with Officer Jones, safe and loved in my new life.

But that wasn't what happened. There were no drugs in the house, the sheriff would tell me the next day, only residue and signs of what had been there. My mother had taken the pipe and the weed with her to Denver. There was nothing to find. And now my parents were on their way home to find out what I had done and begin to clean up the mess. I imagined them seeing the house torn apart. A feeling of fear settled over me, dark and heavy, knowing that things had already changed and I couldn't go back.

The next day, Friday, I sat through each class, watching the clock move closer to three. I anxiously rubbed my thumb in my opposite palm, dispatching my nervousness by pushing harder and harder until my palm was red and raw. Officer Jones came into the cafeteria and found me at lunch. He asked me to go for a walk with him. I was relieved he was here to get me. My stomach had been aching with little pulses of adrenaline all morning, making my mouth dry and sticky and my hands wet and shaky. I felt the hot blood rising in my cheeks and then running cold down my back in a roller coaster of panic and anticipation. When he asked how I was doing, I answered, "Three hours, fourteen minutes. That is all I have. And then it is over. They are going to kill me."

They are going to kill me. It was a juvenile phrase, probably spoken by all children about their parents at some point. But when Officer Jones heard it, he acted swiftly. "Do you think they will hurt you?" He looked at me directly with his dark brown eyes, willing my answer forward with the slightest raise of his brow. "Really?"

I paused and swallowed, wanting to do the right thing somewhere in my life. My actions had set something into motion and it was whirling around me so fast, I could no longer control it. I wanted him to want to love and protect me. "Yes. Really," I replied, turning my eyes down as another flush of adrenaline spiked through my gut. I imagined saying yes would cause Officer Jones to sweep me up in his arms and take me out of my life and into a life with him. I imagined saying yes would make my life better.

I couldn't have imagined what it really meant. What it really meant was a social worker named Jane coming to pick me up from school an hour before the day ended. She would confirm that I felt unsafe, and I would be whisked to a neighboring town and a foster home. My parents would be arrested on their return. It was no longer about drugs. Now it was about child abuse, because I had said I feared for my life.

I was twelve by that time, and almost six months had passed since I met Officer Jones and began crafting my fantasy of freedom into a plan. What I didn't know was that the law wouldn't find enough reasons to remove me from my parents' home permanently. Our lives would go on as they had before, but tainted with the stain of betrayal. I had betrayed them. I selfishly stole the life they had spent so many years building. It was something they would never forgive me for. My family would never be a family again, because of me.

When my family came together for the first time after this, sitting around a small, round table with all four of us and Jane the social worker, my sister kept her eyes down and hugged each of my parents as they cried. I sat alone and silent, at the same table but not with them at all.

"Why would you do this? Why would you lie? What did I do . . . for you to hate me so much?" My mother spoke in broken sentences as tears rushed down her face and my sister leaned closer to hug her. I kept my eyes fixed on the wall ahead. I had no words and certainly no tears left. I sealed up my heart with an iron wall and refused to let their emotions affect me.

My dad spoke in a calm whisper. "We love you, Turtle. We always have. We are here for you." I clenched my gut to keep his words from seeping in. I didn't want his love right now. I wanted to be free and with Officer Jones.

But in the aftermath of my family implosion, he had moved on. He stopped working at the school and disappeared from my life nearly as quickly as he had arrived. And I was left with this table and all the questions about why I would do something so horrible and why what I had was never enough.

The social worker encouraged us to take small steps and be patient as we returned home. We would be required to attend court-ordered family counseling, but after the first session, I was the only one who went back, making it clear that I was the problem. After months of visits, my mother finally came with me again to demand the therapist tell her what I was saying, what further lies I was telling. The therapist refused. "I cannot share with you what she says, I am sorry." And with those words I was whisked away and held prisoner in my parents' home. Soon we packed up and moved to a remote corner of Montana, for a new start.

"I am only taking you with us because the law says I have to," my mother informed me. The irony of her desire to follow this law but not others stung. I heard her clearly—we don't want you; we are forced to take you.

I called Officer Jones on the phone just before we left, hoping I could convince him to rescue me one last time, though I hadn't seen him in months. After my parents' arrest, they took me out of the school on the reservation and drove me to a town fifteen miles away each day. I occasionally saw his truck driving through town, and it would make my stomach drop. I kept hope that he still loved me, like he had promised he always would. When I called, I hoped to remind him of his promise to always take care of me. "This is Melissa," I said softly when he answered the phone. "And I am moving. Leaving forever." I paused, waiting for rescue.

His words came quick and terse. "You cannot call me anymore. Goodbye." And he hung up.

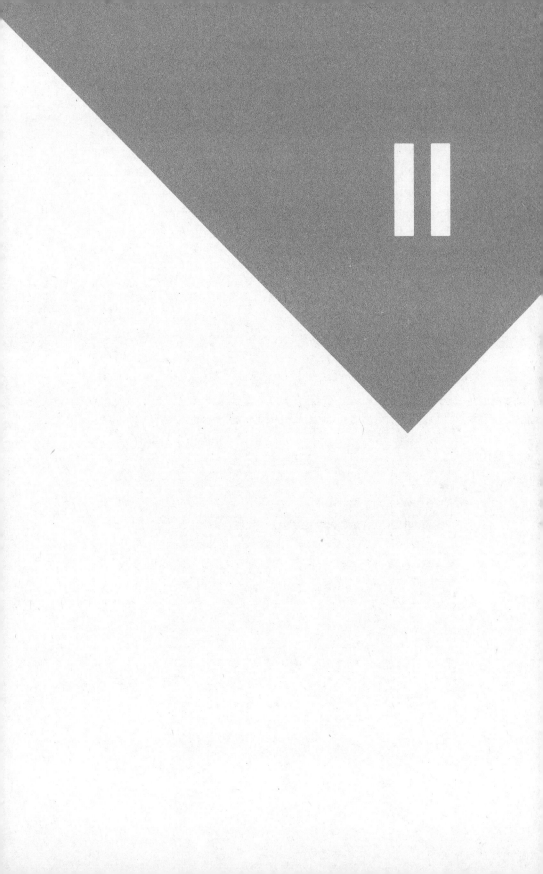

II

4.

SOUL JOURNEY

2002: Northwest Montana

The first rays of the early summer morning sun pushed through the side window of the canopy on the back of my pickup truck, hazy and warm. My truck was providing me a temporary home since I had come back to Montana. I had outfitted it with a little wooden platform made out of plywood to sleep on, and a drawer underneath to store my water jug and camp stove. I used a full laundry bag as a pillow and draped myself with my dad's old down sleeping bag each night. I didn't know how long this would be my home, but I loved the nomadic feeling of being able to park anywhere and have all that I needed. At almost twenty years old, I found that living out of the back of my truck gave me the exact type of freedom I had craved as a child. I was free to go where I wanted, do anything I desired, and be who I wanted to be.[*]

---

[*] Or at least I could pretend to be who I wanted to be as long as it didn't cost any money, because my freedom didn't include anything that exceeded the small sum of money I had saved by working two jobs.

That was what I had come back to Montana for—to find out who I was meant to be. Today marked another promising and terrifying venture toward that goal. I had been invited by my new boyfriend, Gabe, to join a climb up the Great Northern, a mountain that was part of the Flathead range, kissing the edge of Glacier National Park. The Great Northern was a real mountain, rising almost nine thousand jagged, rocky feet from the forest floor right through the tree line and up to the sky. The idea filled me with fear. What if I was too slow, or otherwise incapable? What if I didn't have the right shoes, socks, or sunglasses? But I had washed away my fear with curiosity. What if doing the thing that scared me had the ability to change my life? What if I *could* keep up? My excitement swelled until it was bigger than the fear, and I resigned to keep my own promise to try everything on to see what fit.

I found myself back in Montana because in the three years since I had left, nothing had fit or felt totally right. When I drove away at seventeen, I had been sure I would never return. The timing and horrible circumstances of our move from Colorado had felt like torture to my young teenage self. I was only thirteen when we moved, and being a new girl in a small high school was hard enough, but within the first weeks of school I quickly realized that my Payless sneakers and threadbare Kmart jeans made me an easy target for the polished popular girls who seemed to revel in reminding me that I didn't belong. The boys paid attention to me because I was new, and when I leaned in to that familiar feeling of being wanted by boys, I drew further ire from the girls.

Home was worse. The enraged mother bear was now even angrier, because I had destroyed her den and forced her to move. When I didn't make it home by curfew, I was reminded that I was deceitful and worthless. When I struggled at school and got in trouble for fighting one of the popular girls, she told me it was what I deserved, and that she would kick my ass, too, if she could. I tried on different versions of who I might grow up to be, but none of them fit. I wasn't sporty enough to hang out with the soccer players, nor trendy enough to fit in with the popular girls. I wasn't smart enough to be a nerd. I was just floating in space, a high school girl who didn't fit in anywhere, except with the boys.

I flirted and wore a short skirt, noticing that I was getting noticed, particularly by the older boys. They allowed me to ride in their trucks and attend their parties, but they often expected more than a kiss and so, to keep my place, I obliged and tried to ignore the feeling of being used. I always had a boyfriend and moved quickly from relationship to relationship. The girls who were mean to me as a new kid in school in eighth grade were far more vicious in high school. They wrote "WHORE" on my locker and spread rumors that I was having sex with the teachers. They egged my house and guarded their desks and tables when I came looking for a place to sit. Feeling rejected started to feel like what I deserved. As I approached adulthood, I didn't feel like I could survive much longer in the life I had created. Feeling like I was fighting for my survival at home and in school had become too much. I was a caged animal, destructive in my captivity.

When I did escape, it wasn't in a red convertible or thanks to a dashing savior. Just past my seventeenth birthday, I packed my things into the back of my 1991 black Nissan pickup and left under my own power. I quit high school during my junior year, having negotiated an early exit with both the school and my parents, and eventually I was set free with a GED and a skeptical "Good luck."* I saved money by working the front desk of a health club, cleaning hotel rooms, and babysitting. I tucked twenty-dollar bills neatly together until I had two thousand dollars, the amount I was sure was enough to fund my freedom.

First I went to Oregon, attempting to find work while sleeping on

---

* This negotiation included signing myself out of school under the premise that I was moving. It worked until my biology teacher, ever skeptical of things I said, called the office to ask if my parents had signed me out as well. They had not. My mother was angry, hoping to keep me under her control a while longer. My father was defeated, seeing that I wouldn't survive if I stayed. So they worked with the school to rearrange credits and I took the GED test in exchange for a legitimate exit to my high school days, thankfully.

the couch of my old neighbor from Montana. She was a single mom and an artist who painted pictures of women running naked into the sea, fully themselves, fully authentic. She encouraged me to wade through my teenage sadness and find my authentic self, whoever that was. She gave me a book on tape about the gifts of a wounded childhood. I had spent so many years hearing that I was a liar and a thief, that I was unwanted. I didn't want any of that to be true, but I had nothing to replace it with. I scanned the world for some version of myself that I could sink into. I wanted my authentic self to be someone who would go to college in Portland and live in a cute little apartment while working a quaint little job to support myself. I wanted to be a character in a rom-com, unweighted by my own trauma.

But I was still only seventeen, which made getting a proper job and signing a lease challenging. After I watched my two thousand dollars trickle away without any prospects of replenishment, I packed my truck again and followed a winter fling east to Iowa, where, he told me, I could easily find work. He was going to college there and I would fit right in in his college town, he promised. I figured maybe my authentic self was in the plains of Iowa. I would go and try on a version I hadn't yet imagined, seeing if it fit.

Iowa did have a job for me, working at the front desk of another health club. It had the promise of college on a sprawling and beautiful campus and a cute studio apartment that was my very own.* But no matter how hard I tried to make this life make sense, my authentic self just wouldn't show up. I was doing all the things I had decided to do, but deep down I just didn't feel like myself. I was afraid that who I truly was might be someone that nobody liked, so I kept trying version after version of other people's lives. I absorbed the personalities of the people around me: my boyfriend, his roommates, my co-workers at the health club. I felt like a fraud as I tried to morph myself into the people I was

---

* It was my own, but with the deposit and first and last months' rent paid for by my all-American boyfriend's trust fund, much to my disdain.

close to. But I couldn't shake the person I was underneath, the person who was hurt and trying to protect herself. I wanted to just take on a whole new life and forget my past. I read a book about finding your soul journey and wondered if I would ever find mine.

Then, one day, a co-worker at the running shop where I worked evenings offered me a completely different view on the place I had fled.

"I grew up here." He motioned out into the Iowa night. "And all I wanted to do was go west and climb the mountains. Finally I got a chance, and my friend and I headed to Montana." I heard the way he said the name and even his tone said that it was a wild place. A good place. A place where people wanted to go. "We climbed in Glacier National Park, as many peaks as we could." I listened as he detailed his experiences, both good and bad. I tried to imagine myself in his shoes, scaling the side of a mountain swinging an ice axe. I had promised myself I would never return to Montana, but as he spoke, little flutters of curiosity started to move around my belly. He was envious that I had been lucky enough to grow up in Colorado and Montana. I had never considered that the place I had tried so desperately to flee would be the place someone else would run toward. I had a faint memory of the mountains and the freedom of the outdoors providing me joy as a kid, before I lost sight of all joy and the circumstances of my life began to close around me. Hearing about adventures and independence and exploration made the idea of the mountains seem wild and magnetic again.

With the first spark of inspiration, I shed the life that I was pretending was my own in Iowa and again headed west. I wasn't running from something like when I left Montana the first time; now I was running toward something. John Muir quotes invited me to go get the mountains' good tidings, and I reveled in the romantic notion that somehow mountains could be my home again. Maybe my authentic self had been there all along.

* * *

My little camp stove balanced on the open tailgate of my truck and heated the water for my breakfast. I dug out the old green Gregory backpack that was more of a book bag than a hiking pack. I pulled out my dark gray hiking shoes and a pair of green Old Navy shorts. I cozied into a black Patagonia fleece that I had shoplifted from a local outdoors store while I was in high school. I pushed a headband back to tame my loose hairs, wishing it could tame my anxiety of the unknown, too. As the Montana sun crept up and warmed my body, I felt the unexpected possibility of belonging beginning to take root. Lots of people wanted to climb mountains, and since hearing my co-worker's stories of adventure and freedom, I was one of those people. But first I would have to actually climb one. And not just any mountain—the Great Northern.

The climb would be with Gabe, his parents, and their friends. I had met Gabe not long after arriving back in Montana. He was friends with my high school best friend and I quickly understood that he was *the guy* of their group. He was tan and smart, on break from Harvard and the sailing team he captained. I wanted to be close to him and the great wide world he had access to.

For as much as this Great Northern climb scared me, I thought it was manageable, primarily because we were hiking with his parents and some of their friends. I thought that if people in their sixties were doing this hike, it would be no big deal for me because I had always stayed in shape. I exercised at the gyms I worked at. I ran for an hour each day. And since I had persisted and survived through so much already, how hard could climbing a mountain even be?

I was disabused of my simple notions the moment we gathered. The six older adult hikers were all athletic and muscular, not the shuffling elders I had expected to see. They had bandanas on their necks and sun hats on their heads. Their hiking boots were well worn and told the story of their experience. Gabe and I were the "kids," but Gabe had grown up doing this every weekend. Little waves of nervous nausea started to crash over me as I realized I was out of my depth.

As the ascent began, I stayed near the back, talking with Gabe's dad.

His pace was a steady one that I could keep up with. "You grew up around here, right?" he asked, his voice betraying no exertion.

I was already panting and out of rhythm. "Yeah . . . I could see . . . this peak from my bedroom . . . window." My words came out in short gasps.

I escaped by pushing ahead quickly, lunging straight up the steep forested path and then stopping, gulping the air as he caught up to me and casually continued without so much as a labored exhale. "That must have been beautiful."

After what seemed like a proper eternity, we reached a stunning wide-open meadow. The tall grasses were lush and varying shades of lime, with little wildflowers growing close to the ground. The trees were far below us, and from the perch in the alpine grass, we could see the Bob Marshall Wilderness as it blanketed the landscape, dark and ominous, full of grizzly bears. My face was red and hot, and sweat trickled past my ears, soaking into my headband. Everyone lounged about casually, eating sandwiches and laughing. I was still too nervous and excited to laugh with any ease. Gabe handed me his water bottle. "Here, drink this. The next section is all scrambling!" He sounded excited. I did not know what "scrambling" meant but I nodded, trying not to reveal my ignorance.

The altitude was noticeable now that we were above 8,000 feet. Every part of my body was tired. I thought about heading back down and avoiding all the unknown that was ahead. I began to scrounge around in my mind for an acceptable excuse to leave. Gabe handed me half a sandwich and let his fingers brush mine with a wink. "Are you enjoying this?"

"Totally." I spoke quickly with a little smile, both lying and telling the truth. On the one hand, being here made me want to cry tears of joy. I was actually doing it. I said I was going to do it, and here I was— *doing it.* But I also was physically exhausted from my inefficiency. I was mentally tired from pretending to know where we were and from trying to understand why going slow meant we would get there faster. I watched Gabe interact lovingly with his parents and thought about what my own parents were doing. Their house was just a few hours from here. I had mostly kept my distance from them since I left Montana and had seen them only briefly since I returned. I was a stranger to them now, and I wondered what they would think of me up here, high on the mountain, carried by my own legs.

As Gabe packed his things away and traipsed off, I quickly stood and willed myself to keep up. The meadow gave way to a gentle hill that was less steep than the forest we had already ascended. My calves burned as I attempted to catch Gabe. He was surefooted and unbothered by the altitude. His legs were muscular and with each step his calves would flex and grow, holding his body perfectly steady, never even a slip. His hands were strong from handling the ropes while on the sailing team at Harvard, and when the slope steepened and a wall of rock appeared, he gripped it tightly with those strong hands and pulled his body over the boulders with ease. I was envious, observing his every move, doing my best to mimic him. This, I learned, was scrambling, a marriage of hiking and climbing. The faint trail meandered to the right before jutting up and into the sky, turning from a green meadow path into a knife-edge ridge. The plants faded into rocky alpine terrain and the "trail" became a series of rock steps with the earth falling hundreds of feet on either side of us.

As soon as my shoes touched the rocky ridge, a pulse of excitement shot through my body like a bolt of electricity. Energy flowed up from the ground, through the soles of my shoes, and into my very soul. The thin air somehow started to drench my lungs and nourish my body more than sea-level air ever had. Tears rose in my throat. I was changing the story of who I was from a person who wanted to climb mountains into someone who climbed them. I continued up into the thinner air and the world I had known before began falling away. As we jogged and hopped along the ridge toward the summit, I looked out at the glacier peaks and ridges and saw the promise of unending possibility. I was here, and the rewards I was getting were all because of my own work. I did this myself because doing this was something I was capable of. For the first time in my life, I didn't feel tethered to anything. I was at the very top of my first-ever summit—of a real mountain! As I looked at the land far below me, the place I came from, I had the distinct feeling that anything was possible. If I could do this, I could do anything. I wanted it all. I felt greedy and humbled at the same time. My body was vibrating with the electricity of seeing a version of myself that felt like who I was always meant to be but had never believed I could be.

I soaked it all in until it was time to go down. I wanted to stay forever. That night, I curled into my truck bed and had a dream that I was riding an escalator to the summit of Everest. On top there was a giant pot of soup and people stirring it. I asked them if it counted that I was on the summit since I took the escalator. They told me everything counts, and it does not matter what path you take to get there; you are there. You belong.

* * *

The next months were a series of waypoints on the map I was drawing for myself. It was my first serious attempt to design my own life with the mountains as my guiding light. I would stay in Montana. I would let go of Gabe and stop trying to absorb his life and make it my own. Instead, I spent time trying to form my own identity as a serious climber and hiker and outdoorsy girl. I used my remaining money to sign up for courses in emergency medicine and wilderness medicine. I wanted to feel like a more valuable member of any climbing team I might be lucky enough to join. I bought my first climbing rope and made a list of all the other items I would need. I didn't feel like I was pretending to be someone else, but rather slowly becoming who I needed to be to reach for my dreams. It was a new feeling, one I relished. I read *Eiger Dreams* by Jon Krakauer and fell into a deep fantasy about climbing the biggest mountains in Alaska, like Krakauer had in his twenties. Once again, I worked two jobs to piece together enough to buy one item of gear each month and enough fuel to drive into the mountains at every free chance.

And I started dating Noah. He was my wilderness medicine instructor and the first real-life mountain guide I had ever met. He was short and strong with a thick head of dusty brown hair and a neatly groomed beard. He had straight teeth and curious brown eyes tucked into the weathered face of someone who grew up outdoors. Climbing mountains was his job, alongside teaching wilderness medicine. On our first outing together, we visited a rock-climbing area and he waited patiently while my unskilled hands coiled the rope. With the deft hand of a guide, he adjusted my harness so it was correct without making me feel like it was something I should have already known.* "You are such a fast learner. You are so strong." He encouraged me to push myself harder and learn more. It felt easeful to engage in this relationship with my teacher, and I quickly immersed myself deep into his life. I shared my past with him, telling him about my preteen days as we lay intertwined together in the darkness of a room. He held my secrets gently and expressed feeling guilty that his upbringing had been so untarnished. He didn't treat me like I was broken, and I appreciated that; I wanted to be seen as whole even if it didn't feel totally true.

Noah taught me how to climb multiple pitches of ice with a heavy backpack, and how to plan a day trip with a map and compass. He let me borrow his old, dull crampons and welcomed me into his community of real-life climbers. He guided my first climb of Mount Rainier while letting me believe I was a climbing partner and not simply a student. Unlike the Great Northern, Rainier wasn't a hike; it was a climb. At 14,411 feet above sea level, it is one of the tallest peaks outside of Alaska. Nearly every prolific American mountaineer started out training and climbing there. It was my first big mountain, and I prepared for the climb all summer, carrying water jugs in my backpack up the steep grassy slopes outside of town and reading *Mountaineering: Freedom of the Hills,* the mountain climbers' instruction manual and bible. We would

---

* It was.

be navigating big white glaciers with giant crevasses forming deep cracks. We would be roped together, and I would have to tie all the knots myself. I willed myself to be ready.

And I was, because I had dedicated every waking minute to learning the language of the mountains and making them my home. It wasn't just about mastering the skills of tying knots and handling ropes; it was about self-sufficiency and survival. It wasn't only navigation with a map and compass; it was navigating how to be both a leader and a follower. I read the books and then went out and climbed every pitch of ice I could scratch my way up. I went on my first rock-climbing trips and learned how to lead the rope myself. I practiced rescue scenarios at home, blindfolding myself and running my hands under cold water to mimic the stress of working the ropes during a real mountain rescue. I humbled myself to all that I didn't know and absorbed every experience, letting it shape who I was becoming. I could feel it—this was my path. This was the soul journey that I had read about years before. I was on it, and I had to keep going.

My relationship with Noah was easy and full of fun. He was living the life I wanted to live, and being close to him was helping me get nearer to it. In exchange for access to the world he occupied, the world I hoped to live in one day, I gave him affection and adoration. I let him practice his teaching skills on me and I made him feel like the mountain god he wanted to be. I shushed the little voice in my heart that questioned whether I loved him or if I only loved all that he was giving me access to. I couldn't fully understand what romantic love was yet, as I had held love in a transactional light for most of my life. I had loved what someone could do for me, not who they were to me, perhaps because if I opened my heart and let them in, they would see the real me, and the real me was unlovable. Transactional love was safer.

Soon Noah and I moved in together. I even introduced him to my parents, attempting to ease the strain in my relationship with them. I tried not to care that my mom showered him with the attention and affection she had never given me.

One day, after a long climb in the wilderness of Wyoming, Noah told me he thought I should try out to be a guide on Rainier. We had woken up before sunrise and hiked past sleeping bighorn sheep to arrive at the base of a seven-hundred-foot-tall frozen waterfall. As the sun came up, we used ropes and ice screws to climb up the temporary pillar of frozen water until we reached the top and began the long rappel down to solid ground. It was cold and challenging and beautiful all at once. "Have you thought about guide tryouts?" He asked the question casually as we put away the gear from the day.

"What do you mean?" I looked at him, my very soul illuminated by his words, hoping he meant that I might be good enough.

"You could apply. If you get accepted, you could go try out and come be a guide on Rainier. With me." He might have been asking me because it meant that we could spend our summers together instead of apart. Or maybe he actually thought I was good enough to be a mountain guide. I desperately wanted to be good enough to be a mountain guide. I also wanted to let go of the idea that had slowly taken root during my young adult life that I was wanted *only* as a romantic partner, that my worth was in my body and not in my skills and knowledge.

I thought about the way I had felt standing on the summit of the Great Northern with Gabe, and how far I had come on the journey to find who I was meant to be. Standing on the summits, I felt powerful and capable. I wanted that feeling to last forever. I felt giddy butterflies flapping around in my belly at the thought that all the work I had done had led me here. And I could go even further. Noah believed in me, and I believed in me too. The mountains represented possibilities and freedom, and it was my turn to embrace both.

5.

TRYING TIMES

2004: Mount Rainier, Washington

The rain drizzled persistently on the metal roof, creating a steady and subtle soundtrack to my anxiety. The crowd of people surrounding me, mostly men, were all here for the same reason I was: We were all wannabe guides, lined up for the group tryouts on Mount Rainier. I made sure to keep my face relaxed and soft, not making eye contact with anyone for fear that they might decide that I didn't belong. I stood a little straighter, hoping to create the illusion of a bigger person. What did these sixty people know? How much better and more experienced than me were they? My eyes strained to see through their crunchy new Patagonia jackets and facial stubble.

I had intentionally avoided scenarios like this for most of my life. I was a fast learner but bad at receiving criticism, especially in front of others, which reminded me of being reprimanded by my mother. But I wanted this. More than that, I needed it. One year earlier, just before my twenty-first birthday and days after Noah had suggested I go to tryouts,

I had stood in the bathroom of my tiny cottage house[*] and investigated the eyes looking back at me from the mirror, saying out loud, "I am a mountain guide." It felt good. It felt powerful. It felt different from the previous year of being a student, and a novice one at that.

Since my first steps onto a summit with Gabe, the mountains had felt like home to me.[†] They felt somehow both filled with infinite possibilities and perfectly present. They felt like a place where I could try and fail and I would still be welcomed back to try again. No matter how difficult, unrelenting, or challenging a climb was, climbing had provided me a classroom of endless learning free from the critique of a human teacher. This way of learning was my true north in the crazy bouncing compass of life. Learning was the food that my greedy curiosity craved to satiate it. The more I engulfed myself in learning something new, the more alive and comfortable I felt. Each bit of new knowledge dissolved the bonds that kept me reliant on anyone else. Knowledge was independence, and independence was freedom.

I knew that in the mountains I could never become the master; nature would always have more to teach me, and that thought was intoxicating. Nature could be my mother, firm and unrelenting in her lessons but also warm and cradling, and indifferent to my imperfections—she would hold me regardless of how flawed I turned out to be. These feelings were powerful enough to have pulled me through many moments of discomfort, failing, and flailing to get to this day—guide tryouts on Mount Rainier.

It felt somewhat arrogant to think that after only a year of climbing myself, I could now teach others. I knew that I still had so much learn-

---

[*] Really the shed in the back of someone else's house that had been turned into living quarters for someone who didn't mind a strong draft seeping in during the winter and sharing the kitchen drawers with herds of mice the rest of the year.

[†] Not so much like *my* home, but more like what I thought home should feel like. Cozy and comfortable—a place where you could be messy and vulnerable and know you are still loved. The home I had read about and seen on TV.

ing to do, and if I could somehow convince the people who decide such things that I was a suitable candidate, I would be able to immerse myself in experiences that could make me into who I hoped to become. If I could be a mountain guide, I could be respected. I had seen other girls climbing with their boyfriends and I had heard the whispers about them only being there because their partners climbed. I didn't want to be one of those girls. I wanted respect and power, and the guides had it, undeniably. I could hold the power and people would admire me. They might even love me. I tried on the confidence and esteem of saying out loud what I wanted, and in that minute, I knew that I needed it. It would be worth the fear and discomfort of standing in front of others and showing all that I might not know.

It was the first week of May, and Rainier was still in hibernation. Her slopes had not awakened and avalanched off the grogginess of a winter respite. Climbers were still scarce, so it was the perfect time to invite sixty candidates to a two-day evaluation/job interview/torture-fest. Out of that huge group, the powers that be would wring out the best talent, maybe five or six, and proceed to groom them into brand-new shiny mountain guides who would spend their summer climbing the mountain. The new guides would lead paying clients over the arduous and unforgiving angles of this majestic peak. If you were chosen as one of the few, you would get to wear a stiff red Mountain Hardwear soft-shell jacket with the word "GUIDE" clearly printed on the chest in blocky white letters. I had seen the respect Noah got when he introduced himself as a mountain guide. I craved the same. You were the leader, the keeper of safety, the storyteller, and the strong one. The jacket might as well have said "GOD," because that was the prestige that those who wore it carried.

I wanted to be a god too,* so here I stood on this drizzly morning, worrying if the drizzle was turning to snow up higher and how much

---

* What is the difference between God and a mountain guide? God does not think he is a mountain guide.

faster than me all these boys were going to be. And what about the girls? There were only a few, and the person who was garnering the most attention was not even wearing a Gore-Tex jacket and oversize watch—the standard mountain guide costume. She wasn't even wearing a full shirt. She stood under the propane heaters and the metal awning, casually, with her olive skin and butt-length black hair flowing in shiny cascades around her dark eyes and her tank-top—she was wearing a tank-top! I adjusted my glacier glasses on my head, holding my own short and non-lustrous hair out of my face.

Already in my time on the mountain I had learned how it worked. And apparently, the beautiful dark-haired girl in the tank-top was aware of this as well. This was a man's world and the men made the rules. And according to those rules, as I had watched them play out, it felt like there was only room for one of us, which immediately made her my competition. This was not a new dynamic for me, but rather the continuation of an old one. When it came to men and women, the climbing world intensified the lesson I had internalized from a childhood feeling—like I was competing with my own mother.

I looked down at my well-worn Patagonia* soft-shell jacket with the little black stains—aluminum dust that had been stripped from carabiners by the rope and then transferred permanently to my jacket during a rappel. It made my torso tense with the self-conscious thought that I was not tidy enough for this strange form of a job interview.

The National Park allowed only one service to sell guided climbs of the mountain, and that service bestowed only eighty guides the privilege of taking clients to the summit. I had been told that there were two hundred applicants each year and they whittled it down to this sixty, and at the end of today only forty would remain. That sort of reviewing

---

* I would like to thank Patagonia for choosing Dillon, Montana, to put one of their two outlet stores and for having a sale twice a year that allowed a poor, ramen-eating twenty-one-year-old like me to own and wear their fancy brand and fool the others into thinking I had money too. Thank you, Yvon.

and reduction process made me feel like someone was standing next to me, threatening to tickle me—muscles clenched in anticipation of something that might make me laugh but would also make me uncomfortable.

After what seemed like way too long waiting, the senior guides and supervisors came out to greet me and my anxiety. I noticed the slight shiver of being cold and nervous at the same time—a rigid chill that originates from your center and moves out to your toes and nose. Peter Whittaker stood in front of the group, tall with flowing brown hair and excessively white teeth. He looked like Tom Cruise, but taller. The way he stood with his shoulders relaxed told me that he had all the power, and he knew it. This was Peter's business, handed to him by his father, Lou, a legend of American mountaineering. Lou Whittaker had built Rainier Mountaineering, the largest guide service in North America, after his twin brother, Jim, became the first American to summit Everest.[*]

Peter introduced himself and the cadre of other mountain gods who would decide our fate. They were guides, supervisors, and company owners who had spent years perfecting the craft of a life in the mountains. They knew what they were looking for, and I hoped it was me. After a brief introduction to the gods and the plan for the day, the "mic" was passed over to the sixty wannabes. "Anybody want to step up and introduce themselves?"

I quickly stood, following their directions and giving my designated number first. "Number two—Hi, everyone, I'm Melissa Arnot." I stood as tall as I could—head up, shoulders back, hips forward, stay relaxed (an old running mantra that I found helpful for projecting calm confi-

---

[*] In the pain of competition and comparison that plagues the life of twins, and especially identical twins such as Jim and Lou Whittaker, Jim would rise to the top, making history as the first American to stand on the summit of Mount Everest in 1963. Lou would strive to make his mark, doing many great things and leading a number of expeditions, but he would forever live in second place to the celebrity of his brother. And he would cast the same shadow over his son, Peter.

dence). "I came here from Montana, where I work as an EMT and teach wilderness medicine. I am excited to spend some time outside with you all over the next few days, and hopefully a lot longer than that. Number two."

Peter flashed his bright white teeth at me. "Thanks, Melissa." He made eye contact and smiled at me directly as he spoke my name. The way he spoke to me so directly made me feel both excited and nervous.

Joel, Rob, another Rob, Billy, Jason, Mark, Peter, Paul, another Rob. I sat through the introductions, silently going through crevasse rescue systems in my head and trying to memorize all the supervisors' names. I was looking them up and down and thinking how power can make awkward people look beautiful. I tried to imagine each of them as a waiter or mechanic. Would they look so large and mystical with an apron instead of a harness? Maya—that was Tank-Top Girl's name. She was a BASE jumper and a badass. I took a breath, knowing that she was probably already hired. I silenced the little anger in my gut and reminded myself: skills, leadership, and patience. The mountain does not care if you're cute and busty and brave enough to wear a tank-top to a job interview in the mountains in May. The mountain doesn't follow the rules made by the man.

But the mountain wasn't deciding who got hired, and the people who got hired would be the ones to get to know the mountain. I didn't want it to be true that Maya was taking advantage of the same tools I would use. A flirty smile, a suggestive touch, a tight-fitting shirt. I felt my own shame rise that I had also used my femininity to get ahead, just as I was judging her for doing. I wanted to be seen for my skills and nothing else, but I wasn't willing to let go of some of the practices I knew would work to get me noticed. I wanted to be noticed as Melissa, a new guide candidate who was skilled and passionate and going to do great. Nothing more.

But it wasn't so simple. I had come to these tryouts by way of Noah and his recommendation, and Noah had guided with Rainier Mountaineering Incorporated, or RMI, for years. He had shown me the guide

training manual, told me what guides taught in climbing schools, introduced me to crevasse rescue scenarios, and pushed me to increase my
uphill fitness. He had let me pepper him with questions prior to the tryouts, and most important, he told me I was ready, giving me the boost
of confidence I needed to stand tall in the face of so much unknown. I
had no point of reference for what "ready" was, but he who knew what
they were looking for told me I was perfect. He wanted me to have
everything.

But he did not know that everything included taking a part of him
with me. He had put a small silver ring on my hand the previous fall—I
asked if it meant he wanted to get married, and though he said yes, he
had also never told another person about it, to my knowledge. I imagine
that he had a romantic thought that we would be this couple who could
guide and travel and climb together. And if I had loved him, that would
have been true. But to love meant being vulnerable, which in turn meant
opening myself to being hurt. I wouldn't, and couldn't, do that. So, even
though I cared immensely for him, I kept my heart guarded.

In the process of inching my way forward in my mountain knowledge, aided enormously by Noah and his generosity, I had decided I
would have to leave him behind. The decision was subconscious at first.
It manifested as a slight discomfort at his touch and a deep craving for
my own space. In the months before guide tryouts, I had started spending nights in a sleeping bag, his sleeping bag, on the living room floor of
the little cottage we shared. I said it was because I wanted to wake up
early and train, but really it was because I desperately needed a cocoon
of my own. I was growing little wings and dancing on the edge of the
cliff that would launch me into a creature that could fly, and I saw him
as a weight on my ankle, even though he was the one who had brought
me to this cliff and told me about flying. As long as I was with him, I
knew that I would never be seen as an individual. The questions would
always precede me: Is she only here because she is his girlfriend? Does
she deserve to be here?

Just one month shy of guide tryouts, I had reached the apex of my need for space. Even the sleeping bag was not enough. I took a job as an assistant instructor and weekend chaperone of an ongoing wilderness EMT course in Glacier National Park. It was a dream gig for me in so many ways. I would drive the two hours from Missoula to the park and make a little nest for myself in a simple plywood A-frame cabin with no heat and no electricity. I didn't really get to teach much because I was so new to being an EMT, but I did get to be a patient for the students when we ran scenarios, and I got to hang out with them on the weekends, tasked with helping them prep for their upcoming exam. But mostly, I got to escape Noah and be an individual. It was the first course I worked on without him. It felt good and it felt different, and I was intoxicated by the independence and the possibilities, imagining my life without my achievements being attached to him. No matter how grateful I felt for all he had taught me, I craved being seen as capable on my own. I resented that my accomplishments would be absorbed into my relationship status—even if, or especially because, it was true. I was so grateful, truly grateful for the kindness and acceptance he had shown me. But I wanted to not need anything from anyone. I quieted the voice deep inside that said, *You are only here because of him. You are not ready. You are not enough.* I was here, and it was my turn to prove that I belonged. And so Noah would regret bringing me to a place that was his. He would regret writing me a reference. He would regret lending me his boots for my first climbs. And I would wrap all his regret into a Kevlar blanket, impenetrable and invisible, so I would not have to acknowledge or look at it.

* * *

After the group introductions, the gods loaded us into shuttles with ambiguous instructions: "Bring whatever you think you might need." That was all the information given. We were going on a little jaunt to assess fitness and we would end up somewhere to do something and we should bring things to do that thing, but who knew what thing that was? Bring too much and your pack will be heavy, and you will be slow. Bring too little and you will be fast, but you will not have what you need.

We arrived after forty-five minutes of nervous chatter and launched out the door of the bus and into the snow. The supervisors were assembled, looking like kings. As everyone made their way over, Peter flashed those sparkly teeth and said, "Well, here we go. Let's work up a little lather. Doesn't matter who is first, just don't be last." And off he went, running gazelle-like up the mountain with his long legs and partially inherited, but still hard-earned, fitness. We were chasing the gazelle, but we were not the predators on this run, he was. I breathed deep and hoped my mediocrity would not betray me.

The snowy trail was getting trampled down with each boot in front of me. I looked up, already out of rhythm and breathless. We were running single-file, and I could not pass anyone without punching deep into the soft, high snow on the sides of the trail. I could see the front of the line and not the back. That seemed like an okay place, so I committed to keeping it. All the days of riding my road bike on the steepest hills in Missoula and then running up the "M" hill above the university were serving me. I could do this. I kept whispering to myself that I could do this. I needed this job. The others might want it, but I needed it, and I knew from a lesson in second grade that needs are greater than wants. Needs are things you cannot survive without; wants are merely there to keep the surviving bearable.

My movement was steady as I fast-hiked through the snow, occasionally flirting with a step that resembled running. It was the hardest effort I could sustain. I glanced up through my heaves to see the person in front of everyone else—it was Maya. She was not wearing a tank-top anymore, but I did take note of how tiny her backpack was. I hoped she left behind something critical, and I leaned all the way in to Peter's words: *It does not matter if you are first.*

I held my spot in the middle of the pack for the entire forty-five-minute sprint. I got passed by a few Robs and at least one Paul, but I managed to arrive at the designated spot still in the middle of the pack, just where I wanted to be.* My breath was heavy and short as I exhaled, speaking my number, two, as I arrived and dropped my pack. Peter was already casually eating a sandwich and sitting on his own pack in what I had determined was the required mountain guide seated position: legs crossed, thigh tightly over thigh, torso slouched, and leaning slightly forward. It said, "I'm relaxed but not vulnerable."†

We were quickly divided into smaller groups and told to bring our packs with us as we rotated through the supervisors, each one challenging us to teach a different mountain skill. In my first scenario, one of the Robs started teaching the basics of crevasse rescue to the rest of us as we stood around him in a semicircle. He laid out the rope and hammered the long silver snow stakes, called pickets, into the snow. As he began attaching a pulley to the rope, the supervisor abruptly stopped him and tossed the lesson to me. My gut flipped. I was confident in setting up my rescue systems after months of practicing them blindfolded, but Rob was doing it wrong—he'd missed some critical steps right at the top. I panicked inside, my mind quickly entering a college-level debate-team argument over whether to continue without correcting Rob's mistakes or to point them out and fix them. I swallowed hard and stepped up, swiftly dismantling the incorrectly rigged system. "Thanks, Rob. Let us review some of the basics that Rob got us started with. Before you can attach the pulley, what elements does your anchor need to have?" I gently queried my peers, hoping I had gracefully sidestepped this bomb, without calling Rob out but also not letting his mistakes be my founda-

---

* I wanted to be first. But that wasn't possible, so I told myself that I wanted to be in the middle. The middle is the best. Think of an Oreo—what a gross cookie without the middle. Peanut butter and jelly? Just bread without the middle. The middle is what we should all strive for.

† It is the opposite of manspreading, and you do not commonly see men sitting this way, but all the mountain guides do. Once you see it you cannot unsee it, and it made me wonder what they were all protecting.

tion. A different Rob shouted an answer: "Equalized!" "Right," I replied, "and that is where it all starts. Things must be equalized."

The core foundation of a strong anchor in any type of climbing is that it is equalized. There must be more than one point, and each point must share the load equally. It is not negotiable. They not only back each other up but they share the weight before a backup is ever needed. I was in love with the idea that my climbing relationships, and all my relationships, could adhere to this same simple principle. But I quickly learned that things would rarely be equal and only sometimes fair. And that fair and equal have nothing to do with each other.

The show-and-share stations continued in this fashion for half of the day. I carefully observed the way the supervisors set down their packs, what they pulled out of them, and how they moved. They seemed to have a secret language of knowing that none of the wannabes could yet speak. They conveyed emotions to one another even with their eyes masked behind mirrored wraparound glacier glasses. Seeing the gods in their heaven made me want it even more.

Before the day ended, Peter circled everyone up and shared some insight into what guiding meant to him. He sat cross-legged on his backpack in the snow, looking comfortable and at home. "There is no better job. You get paid to do the thing people are paying to do!" he said. "Listen, I grew up watching my pop run up this mountain and drag ropes of clients up. I started following him when I was twelve. And by the time I was twenty-one I was traveling the world and working as a heli-ski guide in Utah." Everyone sat still, enraptured by his ease and likability. He was warm and funny and yet firm and stoic, somehow melting the contradiction into the guy everyone wanted to be around. Every young guide-in-the-making leaned closer to breathe in each word, in case his charisma was contagious.* I wanted to catch it too. I kept my

---

* The age range of the participants at guide tryouts was vast. I was one of the youngest at twenty-one. There were at least two men in their fifties, and most of the population was spotted with mid-twenties to mid-thirties dudes. I came to learn that this was by

eyes on him when he spoke and nodded gently so he would know I heard him since my eyes were covered.

We all shuffled back into the shuttle buses and drove back down to the little logging town that was serving as our base camp for the tryouts. The supervisors were offering us a free night in guide housing bunks if our name appeared on the list of people invited back for a second day. I had already decided that if I made it, I would stay in my truck rather than in the guide housing with my competition. I didn't want to just be one of them; I wanted to be different, better, more. I would be more than happy to find a pullout on an old logging road and tuck myself in with a beer and the drizzle of rain peppering the canopy of my truck.

The list of forty candidates who survived the first cut came out around four p.m., and we all rushed to the wall to find our names. As soon as I saw mine, I scurried away, wanting to quickly get out of there and get some rest. I wanted to let my guard down a little in a way I could not under the watchful eye of the gods. Halfway through the parking lot I turned back to see Maya, the beautiful badass, wiping tears from her face and getting and giving hugs to a small group that surrounded her. I also saw my trekking pole still leaning against the building, offering me the excuse I needed to go look at that list a second time, without the crowd. Sure enough, Maya was not on the list. *Holy shit.* The fastest person on the endurance test, the most beautiful person at the tryout who also happened to be a fearless skydiver, did not make the first cut. I couldn't understand. It did not fit the pattern that I had become accustomed to. The cute girl always got picked. I had seen it work to my own advantage before—if you were a girl in a man's world your best chance of being valued was by being beautiful. But maybe this man's world was different from the ones I had grown up in.

---

design. A supervisor later told me that unmarried thirty-year-old men had a fatalistic view and need to test death, making them perfect for a risky job of tying yourself to total novices and traipsing underneath monolithic ice and rock that cascaded down regularly. I wondered what this said about me.

The second day of tryouts started with a series of skills tests. We were blindfolded and asked to give first aid to a wounded climber, as a team. We were told to build an anchor, and once it was done the supervisor came and took one item, a carabiner or nylon sling, away and told us to do it again with what we had until we couldn't do it anymore. All the supervisors had clipboards and pens, and they made private notes next to our numbers and names.

While I was waiting my turn to build an anchor out of dwindling supplies, the supervisor at that station set down the clipboard with the notes showing. I scanned quickly for my name and number and saw the typed words "MELISSA ARNOT, W-EMT, AVY II, ENGAGED TO NOAH DRIGGS."

I was instantly furious. Right there, next to my credentials, was my relationship status, or my supposed relationship status. I bristled at the fact that Noah had told the supervisors we were engaged, even though he hadn't told his family or mine, and I didn't think we were really engaged. Regardless, I didn't want to be his anything, especially not through the lenses of my potential future bosses. My heartbeat quickened as a hot, angry red flush moved up my neck. I wanted to be judged on my confidence and how I carried myself and on my ability to build an anchor system faster than nearly anyone else. I wanted to be judged because I had hundreds of hours spent caring for sick and injured people in emergency situations, and I had the ability to stay calm under immense stress. But seeing my connection to Noah noted on the clipboard made it feel like all my accomplishments had been erased. This was what I had feared all along: I would never know if I was there because of him or because of the work I had done to be there.

I knew I couldn't just let this go, even if this meant I would lose my chance to be a god too.

The second part of the morning was interviews. Each guide was brought into a room with either multiple guides and one supervisor or multiple supervisors and one guide. It was our chance to be memorable. When my number was called, I walked in to see Peter Whittaker; Lindsey, a second-year guide who was the only woman helping all the male super-visors with the tryouts; and Paul Maier, a supervisor who had been working on the slopes of Rainier for twenty years. Paul was the type of stoic whose hard edges could make a rock look like a pillow. He was emotionless and stern, and I was strangely terrified of him.

Peter spoke first, flashing his mouth pearls in a comfortable grin. "This station is about clients' questions. I am supposed to ask you about layering with cotton. But I just want to tell you, I think you know that we really want to hire you. You are exceptional, the total package." As those words escaped his mouth, I hid my disgust at what I thought that term implied with a gentle smile and a faux shy look at my feet. I breathed deep, knowing that what came next was going to take courage. "So instead of asking you questions, do you have any questions for us?" Here was my chance.

"Well, first, thank you," I replied. "It is hard to know where one stacks up against the others, so I appreciate that you might want to hire me. I would like to say one thing, though."

As I paused, Lindsey jumped in: "Be careful what you say; you are doing good so far." She stared at me as I wondered what kind of advice that was.

I nodded as I inhaled and pressed my lips together. "I just wanted to ask you . . . I wanted to say—if you want to hire me, I want you to hire me based solely on what you have seen here and my résumé, not who I know. I saw the paper said that I am Noah's fiancé, and I am not. We are not together anymore. So if you want to hire me, please make it based on what you've seen over the last two days."

I spoke the words quickly and clearly, with the same confidence with which I had taught ice axe arrest the day before. But as soon as they left my mouth, I shrank into the surprise of what I had just said. I had wanted to say, "Hire me for me! I am good enough without my connec-tions!" But instead, I revealed far too much.

The relief of speaking up and the panic of telling them that Noah and I had broken up before I had actually broken up with him washed over me at the same time, a collision of confusing emotions that threatened to sap my confidence. I willed my shoulders down away from my ears as my body tensed up. *Jesus, why did I have to say that?* What if they deemed it too messy to have me there now? What if someone talked to Noah before I could? I breathed into the moment and swallowed, maintaining my own emotionless facial expression.

Peter Whittaker's mouth pearls seemed to shine even brighter as a big smile crossed his face. "Thank you for saying that. Like I said, you are the total package. Thanks, Melis." I stood to go, feeling weird that Peter Whittaker was already calling me by a cute nickname but relieved that I had not been dismissed summarily.

The day ended early for all the wannabes so the supervisors could deliberate and we could writhe in the discomfort that would come before the knowing. The final, and most important, power that the gods wielded came in the form of the List—the posting of the six names of the newly hired guides and three "cuspers," or alternates, in case one of the six did not stand the test of a climb. That List held even more power, because we were going to be ranked in the order we had performed. I sat on one of the massive wood picnic tables, chatting with the other nervous candidates. People were making tentative plans of where they would stay that night, not knowing if they were going to be invited to stay here or sent home. From the picnic table in the yard, we could see through the glass door of the deliberation room. I wondered what they were debating. I wondered who was being joked about. I wondered what happened to Maya the day before. And then Peter came out holding the results.

"Thanks, everyone, for coming out these last few days. It was great to get to know some of you." *Ouch.* "If your name is on the List, we want to invite you into the guide lounge to have a beer and welcome you to the team. If not, sorry about that, and we encourage you to reach out via email if you want more feedback." The humble white paper that made or broke dreams was tacked onto the wall, and Peter returned to the guide lounge.

I took a deep breath and watched the flurry of wannabes huddle. I told myself to just wait. One of the Robs went into the guide lounge, followed by a Joel. I walked slowly to the List, feeling angry that this paper had so much power and I had none. And there it was. My name. Number one, Melissa Arnot. I was the first pick.

Chills spread like a grass fire over my body, and I tried not to tear up. I had been mediocre at nearly everything I had tried to do in my whole life. My sister was called "Little Miss Perfect" by our sixth-grade teacher, and when I arrived in his class he called me "Little Almost Miss Perfect." I was second born, and I got second place in the spelling bee and the hundred-meter dash. I was supposed to be in the middle. I had never been number one at anything. But here I was, at the top of the list. They were telling me, "We want you the MOST." I felt like it must be a mistake.

I walked into the guide lounge, the hangout of the gods. I smiled and exhaled, trying to get comfortable with the idea that I could now be one of them. My body still felt tense but my mind began to ease with the elation that I had made it through the door. They would teach me their secret language and I would learn the way to sit in the tightly twisted way of the gods. I would get the beautiful letters emblazoned across my chest that said I belonged. I would get to enter the closed doors of the guide lounge, part of a team. I had spent so much of my young life believing that I didn't belong anywhere, but with my name on this paper, I could finally, for a moment, feel a sense of belonging in a family that wanted me.

I sat down next to the medical supervisor, hopeful he would be an ally because of our shared interest in medicine. He shook my hand and handed me a cold white can with red cursive letters, Rainier Beer. "Congratulations," he said while holding up his can for a toast. I relaxed my shoulders and said thank you, tapping my can on his. "So, you're Noah's fiancée?" he asked, adding a condescending smirk that reminded me that I might be in the lounge of the gods, but I still had no power here. No matter what I had said to Peter, Lindsey, and Paul, they still saw me dressed in the costume of Noah's fiancée, a person who didn't earn her way here.

"I was . . ." I started to awkwardly acknowledge, but just then Peter Whittaker stood up and started speaking. I experienced a wash of gratitude to him for unknowingly saving me with his interruption, when suddenly the glass door opened and in walked Maya, looking gorgeous, relaxed, and confident, with her long hair framing her face. My shoulders slumped, confused by this unexpected guest. As far as I was concerned, this was already my place, and anyone without their name on the List was a guest, including her. "Hey, Maya, have a seat," Peter said, pointing to an open spot next to me. "Maya is the most important person in this room," he said, smiling gently her way. What was that supposed to mean? My confusion and anger tangled together. "She's going to be joining us this summer as a cook up at Camp Muir, so be extra kind to her." She grinned and sat down beside me.

My throat filled with a lump as the heat of strong emotions rose up my neck. Did they offer the job of cook to any of the other castoffs, or only to the attractive girl? She couldn't be a guide, but she could be the cook for the guides?* The invisible infrastructure of the house of the gods was starting to reveal itself to me, and even though I didn't like what I saw, I knew I was going to have to reside there. I wondered if I would ruin this house, too.

* * *

After taking the job, I knew one thing remained before I could move forward—the unavoidable task of actually breaking up with Noah. Since I had outed myself to his, and now my, entire workplace, I didn't have the

---

* There is a long and predictable history with cooks on Rainier becoming the mistresses, girlfriends, and wives of the guides, so this role was particularly telling in how her value was perceived. Peter's dad, Lou, had left Peter's mother for a cook, who he later married. And now Maya, the most beautiful girl at the guide tryouts, was being hired to cook for, and presumably be the girlfriend of, the guides. The pattern would repeat itself again and again.

luxury of doing it at a quiet and leisurely pace. I hoped, even imagined, that it would be smooth and easy, that he would understand that we had grown apart. But the truth was that I had grown away from him without ever giving him a sign that it was over. He was in a relationship with my ghost, projected so intentionally that he couldn't even tell I wasn't there.

"I think that we have grown apart and want different things now." I leaned on the edge of the door to the little camper he lived in for the summer while he was guiding. I spoke the words gently, then looked at him, hoping to see him nodding in agreement. Instead, he looked at me with complete shock. He had just returned from Denali, and it was only two weeks since I had been hired.

"You want to break up?"

He was asking a direct question. But I couldn't give him a direct answer. I spent the next months letting him hold on to hope while I said I just needed a little space. It was cruel. I could feel the cruelty of it in the slight kindness he continued to show me. I muted the part of my conscience that was horrified that I was hurting him to continue my path forward at work. I told myself that he was strong and would be okay. And I busied myself with learning the tactical job skills of rescue and climbing and avoided the sticky guilt and shame that lived in my quiet moments.

When I finally did end it, just weeks into my new career as a guide, he was devastated. He passed through the stages of grief in textbook order, starting with denial. I wasn't really done, he told me. I just needed a break, like I had said. When I somehow held my ground, he moved quickly to anger. He made me give him back the boots I had borrowed to start my guiding career, and he sneered at my inexperience. Then came the bargaining—if I would just go on a drive, a climb, a trip with him, we could work this out. If he let me have the summer away, would I come back to us in the fall? I said no, and held the small distance I had scooped out, feeling weaker and more unsure of myself with each phase.

When the despair phase came, I ran. I stopped speaking to him at all and created distance in whatever ways I could. I had spent all of the years since my childhood avoiding the emotional fallout of my actions by running away and neatly packing the other person's feelings into a box I would never open again. This was how I had escaped my family as a teen, how I had hopped from boy to boy in high school, how I had quickly moved from my Iowa boyfriend to Gabe and then on to the next one with little pause between. From then on, when Noah and I crossed paths, I blurred my gaze when I looked his way and continued on, both without him and without acknowledging that I wouldn't even be here without him. I acted like I barely knew him at all and insulated my emotions from his sadness. I wanted to have done it all on my own, but the truth was more complicated than that—so I ignored it and entangled myself in the next thing, never looking back at the mess I left behind.

This, predictably, made things worse. "You might be moving on now. And you think I'm pathetic," he hissed, looking at me with disgust. He was sitting in his truck, speaking to me through the window after finding out I was dating another RMI supervisor. "But trust me, in time this is going to come back, and you are going to be the one to have to deal with it." I told myself he was just hurt and he would surely get over it. I had, so why couldn't he? But he was right. The actions I was quickly moving through while ignoring the consequences would come back and stay with me for far longer than his heartache ever lasted.

6.

CAPTIVITY

2004: Mount Rainier, Washington

After I received my red soft-shell jacket with "GUIDE" printed in all caps on the left front chest, I was given a shared room in a shared house: two women, fourteen men, three bathrooms. My schedule was filled each month with a combination of one-day climbing schools to prepare the clients to climb Mount Rainier, two-day summit climbs, and the occasional longer mountaineering course, typically reserved for guides more senior than me. When there was no space on the schedule for the new guide, I was given a fifty-pound load to carry up to the 10,040-foot-high camp. Each outing was a deluge of learning: learning how to safely encourage brand-new climbers out of their comfort zone; figuring out what each senior guide valued most, your words or your silence.

I had never seen the inner workings of a fraternity, but this was what I imagined it to be like. Dirty dishes left in the kitchen were swiftly transported to the bed of the guide who was thought to have left them there. The most important thing I learned about living in a house with fourteen men was that you NEVER leave your toothbrush in the bathroom. It would get used by whoever needed one, or, worse, it would be covered with specks of discarded facial hair from someone's hasty shave before the morning meeting. I refused to clean up the messes that the guys left around the house. I would not accept the maternal role that they seemed to silently drape on the few girls who were around.

But I heard the whispers and saw the doe-eyed smiles aimed in my direction. The language of flirtation was not foreign to me; rather, it was almost my first language. I had cracked the code at a young age, and in return, I had been given access to spaces where there was power and adventure. From one of my first health club jobs in Montana when I was fifteen, when I had been promoted after spending time flirting with my fifty-six-year-old boss, I had repeated this pattern in job after job. Now I was trying to reverse that, making every attempt to be known as the hardest-working guide on the mountain. But every climb ended at the tavern in town, where the boys' memory of my early wakeup to shovel the path into camp was replaced by how I looked in jeans and a tank-top. And I sipped my beer and smiled straight back at them, especially those who had the power.

What I wanted most at that moment was this job, this life, and the path of adventure and freedom it would take me on. It wasn't just Noah; I created a quick and heartless equation to assess the people around me: If someone wasn't a stepping stone, they were an obstacle. If I didn't allow myself to be fully seen by someone, they couldn't reject me. I would get to be the one to reject them, and after the experiences of my childhood I coveted that role greedily. I discarded human roadblocks without hesitation or consideration of their feelings, hoping they would fade into the background, never to rise again. Noah was a roadblock. My family was a roadblock. I set them aside in a dark corner of my mind and hoped they would never wander back into the light.

The new RMI supervisor I was dating, Brad, had more experience and therefore was a bigger stepping stone than Noah. He was thirty-three,

I was twenty-two. In many ways, he was my boss. I wanted the chance to guide all around the world, and he could offer exactly that. Brad was stoic and stern and committed to climbing like no one I had known before. He had a small, quiet smile and a humility (it seemed) that other guides didn't possess. We started hanging out on our days off from guiding and going rock climbing every chance we had. One afternoon at the local crag we frequented, he handed me the end of the rope and gestured me up first. "You lead this one. Your back and shoulders are so strong. It's incredible to watch you." He gave me one of his quiet smiles as I considered trying to lead one of the hardest climbs I had ever tried. I blushed at his praise and his belief in me. I enjoyed the way his eyes watched me so closely. He cheered me on and made me feel capable. If he believed in me, maybe he was right.

Brad introduced me to clients as one of the best and hardest-working new guides he had ever worked with. As I'd hoped, he told the owners of the company, including Peter, that he wanted me on all his international trips. I found myself attracted to his power and his praise. And also to him. He was muscular and tan with a full head of bright blond hair and crystal-blue eyes. I enjoyed the earliest days of flirtation turning into something more as I imagined all the places this new relationship would take me,* never wanting to acknowledge the relationship for what it was: the next rung on the ladder I was climbing. I was using the men in my life to get what they had, softening them into loving me while I hardened myself to loving them back. Later I learned that some fellow climbers called me a lumberjack—I chopped down the men like trees and left the forest a wreck.

But because the primary equation of my relationships was how they could advance me, not the quality of the partnership, my choices were starting to have consequences. Getting what I wanted required sacrificing myself more and more along the way. Weeks into dating, Brad and

---

* I am the worst, I know.

I went on our first trip together on a three-day break from guiding. It was his birthday and the season was nearing an end. This was our first chance to take our new love out of the confines of the sphere of Rainier. The first thing that struck me like a lightning bolt was his inability to compromise on anything—the route we drove, the music we listened to, or the food we ate. There was only one way, and it was his way.

"Hand me your phone." His words were cool as his eyes stayed on the road while he drove. In the few weeks that we had been officially dating, he had already scrolled through my email account on the computer in the guide lounge. He had rifled through the glove box of my truck and looked closely at how many voicemails I kept stored on my flip phone. When he asked for the phone, I wouldn't hesitate to give it to him, and he would scroll through looking for signs that I was unfaithful or dishonest. Control. I shuddered. It was the thing I had most eagerly fled as a child and now here I was, voluntarily ensnaring myself in it because I believed what I was gaining was more than what I was giving up.

By the time the three days' climbing ended, I had already started to plot our breakup. It would be okay, I told myself, since we hadn't been dating that long. I would have to go back to Montana for the winter and it was doubtful he would join, as I didn't even have a place to live. I would just kind of let our relationship fizzle and that would be the end.

On the drive home he spent five hours quizzing me with the interrogation skills of an FBI agent about our physical relationship. Was I attracted to him? Wasn't this a new relationship and meant to be always physical and always hot? Was I attracted to someone else? When we arrived back at Rainier, I leapt out of the car, finally feeling able to breathe. I went to the guide lounge to see the schedule and found that my remaining climbs of the season were almost all with Brad. There would be no easy fade-out.

As soon as I tried to create space between us, he would dangle his power: *Do you want to guide with me in Ecuador this winter? Do you want to go to Aconcagua with me?* I did want both of those things, and so I found myself in a tortured equation of wanting the opportunity but also wanting my freedom. I knew I could not have both, and so I swallowed the glass of shattered self-value and stayed with him. Maybe this is what I deserved after breaking Noah's heart, I thought.

Over the following months, we rode a volatile roller coaster of mistrust, suspicion, and control—almost ownership, his of me—punctuated by moments of feeling like I was a queen and I could do anything. But those moments would pass quickly and his jealousy would reemerge, causing another outburst and continuing the cycle. Just when I was sure I couldn't possibly stay another minute, Brad would shower me with compliments and praise and lift me higher than I had ever been held. I exchanged the shower of his adoration for the prison of his jealousy. When I stood too close to another male guide or smiled too sweetly at anyone but him, he spiraled into a possessive rage. His unpredictable moods anchored me back to my childhood and the cautious way I approached my mother, unsure of who she might be at any moment. But he was a step to who I so desperately wanted to become, so I swallowed my discontent and reminded myself that discomfort often had a purpose.*

And I got my reward, traveling by Brad's side to Ecuador, my first time climbing and working out of the country. We were picked up at the bustling South American airport by a friend of his. As they spoke to one another in Spanish, I felt ashamed that I didn't know more of the language. I started a notecard that night, writing every Spanish word and phrase I could remember and practicing them again and again. The clients arrived shortly after us and I dutifully shadowed everything Brad did. Most of them he knew pretty well and had courted for this trip. Two older guys and two in their twenties, the latter from whom I kept my distance for fear of angering Brad. We completed multiple hikes in

---

* This is something I spent years feeling ashamed of. I was using him to advance my career and that truth felt disgusting, so I chose not to look too closely at it. I assured myself that it was okay, because of the way he was treating me. But those assurances did little to quell the guilt I felt for not being a better human.

the high, grassy hillsides of Ecuador, and I soaked in the smells and sounds of this foreign place. On the first climb the wind howled through the night as we passed 16,000 feet and then 17,000. It was as high as I had ever climbed, and here I was, guiding. Brad set the pace and found the route, and I followed, trying to memorize each detail. This was the payoff for enduring his unpredictability.

At the end of my first year as a guide on Rainier, I took the series of exams that allowed me to become a lead guide. I passed, and over time I became the Guide, capital G, I had always wanted to be. I was no longer only a follower; I was the leader now, too. Brad praised my rise as he kept a firm hand on my shoulder.

* * *

Early in the spring, after returning from a few weeks climbing in Oregon with Brad, I sat silently in my single-cab dark blue Toyota truck. The chill of a Montana winter was all around, even in March as the spring tried to fight her way in. I turned off the ignition and looked around the storage unit complex as Ani DiFranco played from my truck's weak speakers. I looked at the little blue-and-silver flip phone on my lap, and then at the door of the storage unit—the Sheddy, as it was known. This was part of my job with Aerie Backcountry Medicine. In addition to the fun job of teaching wilderness medical courses, I was bestowed with the unfun job of cleaning, organizing, and packing gear for all of the courses. I spent an unreasonable amount of time at the Sheddy re-rolling gauze bundles after students had stopped fake bleeds in scenarios. I cleaned fake blood from the sleeping bags and coiled the ropes that would be turned into rescue stretchers by the next students. The job was a direct view into the space between an ending and a beginning. It was a putting-back-together of sorts. So it only felt right that I would be sitting here contemplating a phone call I did not want to make, in an attempt to put myself back together.

The phone number was written on a scrap of paper and the phone was in my hand, but I couldn't make the call. I wanted to wish this away. I wanted to just go to sleep and wake up and for everything to have fixed itself. I took the deepest breath my nausea would allow and dialed the number, holding the little phone to my ear and holding my breath until the receptionist answered.

"Planned Parenthood of Missoula."

I wondered for a moment what it was like to answer the phone knowing that someone else's shame and fear and pain were calling you right now. "I want to schedule an abortion." I exhaled.

The receptionist informed me that it would cost $575, payment required up front. I felt the heat of emotion run up my chest and into my throat, and explode out my eyes in scalding tears. "What if I can't pay that?" I asked in a sudden rush of fear. I had no extra money. I wouldn't start guiding again until May, and I was using every last dollar to keep afloat until then. I had no more credit on my credit cards. I had no permanent address and no safety net to borrow money from. I lived in a precarious financial balance that had already been thrown off by having to fix the engine in my truck the previous fall.

"Sell your car, get a loan, use a credit card. There are ways." She said these words to me in a cold and matter-of-fact way. I couldn't sell my car because I needed it to do my job. I felt overwhelmed and alone. I said thank you and hung up.

The tears kept falling as I slinked deeper into the bench seat of the truck. Why was this happening? Why hadn't I broken up with Brad the thousand times that I had wanted to? I knew the answer too well to even ask.

As waves of nausea washed over me, I cleaned up the Sheddy and weighed my options. I would have to tell Brad. He was living in our friend's guest shack in Oregon until guiding started up again. We had just returned from a trip to Aconcagua, our second international guiding trip together, marked by our typical roller coaster of interactions. The start of the trip was loving and encouraging, but by the time we returned to Mendoza, Brad was no longer talking to me unless it was to quietly berate me for how I both talked kindly to the clients and didn't have enough sex with him. We had parted ways after a short time together in Oregon, but we hadn't broken up. He was going to spend some time rock climbing while I worked a few courses and made some more money. We talked on the phone almost every day, but I had been feeling beyond grateful to have some space from him. And now, this.

I decided the best thing I could do was make a plan and ask him to help me execute it. I spent a few hours on the internet that afternoon, scouring for options. Oregon Planned Parenthood had some funding options that I might be able to take advantage of. I called the clinic in the town near where Brad was staying and made an appointment. I called him and told him I was coming to Oregon.

I knew Brad wanted kids badly. I did, too, but one day in the future, and not with him. I didn't want to even tell him I was pregnant for fear of what would happen if I told him I wanted an abortion. But now I was going to have to. I couldn't do it without his financial help, and this truth weighted me down like a shipping container sinking to the bottom of the ocean.

When I got to Oregon, I sat with Brad the first night and summoned the courage to speak. He was staying in a little one-room cabin on his friend's property, close to a rock-climbing area. The room was small and always too cold or far too hot once the small woodstove overheated the space. I sat next to him on the bed, the only furniture in the room, sweating from the heat of the fire. "I have to tell you something." I paused and considered just running out of the room. "I am pregnant. I was taking birth control, so . . . I don't know." I hoped I could somehow leap into my own pause and disappear before he would be able to react. But he met the news with gentle and warm eyes.

"What do you want to do?" he asked kindly. His kindness made me want to cry.

"I feel like I cannot become a parent right now. I have no money. I have no stability."

"Kids are born in far worse situations and it's okay." He offered this as a comfort, but it felt abrasive to my heart. I was born to a mother who didn't want me. I would never repeat that for my own child.

I told him I wanted an abortion, hating myself for even saying those words. He nodded with understanding and offered his support for whatever I wanted. He would pay for half and go with me to the clinic.

His kindness caught me terribly off-guard. But he also spent the week that I had to wait for my appointment telling me what a beautiful pregnant woman he thought I would be. He would mention how he hoped this didn't harm me in a way that I would never be able to have kids in the future. He would talk about how joyful it would be to meet our child one day. His words brutalized me, cruelty disguised as kindness. The torture I felt in my heart was a bleeding wound, and his words were vinegar to it, making sure I felt its pain. At twenty-two, how could I know if this was the right thing? If I never got pregnant again and I never became a mom, this moment and this choice would torture me forever. But at the same time, how could I justify having a child that I knew I was not equipped to take care of? And even worse, what if it was a girl and she was subjected to the same abuse, control, and mental games that her dad subjected me to? Even though the decision was tortured and painful, I knew it was the right one.

The morning of the abortion Brad drove me to the small clinic. I entered the exam room alone and they asked me if I wanted him there. I did not. In fact, I wondered if there was a way they could make him disappear completely. I went back to the waiting room after getting an exam and being given a valium to soften the edge of irreversible choices. I scanned the room. A young teenage girl and a man who appeared to be her father. Two girls in their twenties who looked like they could be friends but clearly didn't know each other. A woman who looked to be forty, with the style and composure of a real estate agent. And me. A flip-flop–wearing mountain guide sitting stiffly next to a boyfriend she did not want. We were all sisters in this. We were all at a junction, and we had all chosen to go right. And now we just had to wait our turn.

The procedure was systematic and shockingly quick. I was sent to another room, partially occupied by my sisters from the waiting room. We were all given juice and crackers and treated like the children we had just opted out of having. When sufficient time had passed and any residual tears had been blotted by the rough and thin industrial tissues of a clinic buying in bulk, we were returned to the waiting room and a world that was certainly different from the one we left just half an hour before. I saw Brad and I realized that I had been partially holding my breath for the past few weeks. I was waiting to see what would happen. And now it was done and I could breathe again.

I nestled myself in the front seat of his old Subaru as we drove back toward his friend's place. He didn't say anything, and his silence made me both grateful and fearful. As we pulled up the gravel driveway, he looked over at me. "You know," he said, his voice almost a whisper but steady, and his eyes fixed, unblinking, on me, "you didn't even ask me what I wanted. You decided to do this yourself. You did not even give me a choice. You never think of us. You are just a selfish bitch." And with that, he turned off the car and went inside.

Brad's words trickled through my ears, that day and many days after. *What if you can never be a mom? You selfish bitch.* I did not want them to stay with me. I wanted to have such a strong sense of self that they did not affect me at all, but it just was not true, and I found myself crying into my shirtsleeves whenever I was alone in my truck. My heart was broken and inside the cracks lived his words, distant threats that I couldn't forget.

7.

FALLING

2006: Mount Rainier, Washington

When the summer season started a few months later, I dedicated myself fully to my work, both the technical, physical aspects, and the soft skills of helping people do really hard things and ushering the vulnerability that requires. In a way, protecting clients' vulnerable selves was saving me from having to expose my own. My clients appreciated my patient and firm leadership. The other guides leaned on me for my medical knowledge when things went wrong. And Peter Whittaker noticed me.

At the end of my second season guiding on Rainier in 2006, Peter asked me to assist him and the celebrity climbing guide Ed Viesturs on their annual Whittaker-Viesturs climb. It was a four-day luxury climb on Rainier with guests paying almost five thousand dollars per spot to ascend in the shadow of climbing fame and celebrity. Ed had just completed climbing the fourteen highest mountains on Earth without the use of supplemental oxygen, an American first and the culmination of a twenty-year project. Meeting him was exciting and intimidating. He was a compact and athletic man with a perfectly V-shaped torso. He had deep lines in his face and he held the stern expression of someone who could get things done. I was nervous to be around someone so accomplished, and I disguised this by asking him how he got to the Himalayas for the first time. He was brief in his explanations but offered me little nuggets of advice. I tried to keep a slight distance from him, unsure what to say.

Peter was charismatic and entertaining. I was there to fill in any gaps that they might need taken care of, which meant I mostly spent my time digging tent platforms, setting the tents up, or fixing the crampons of a client. I watched Peter carefully, trying to guess what he might need and provide it before he asked. Throughout the climb Ed was quiet and stern; he seemed to feel somewhat inconvenienced to be guiding Rainier after all his success. As we lay head to toe in our three-person tent, I listened to them divide the clients for the climb into rope teams. Peter took the strongest, Ed the most "important," and I took the stragglers. If someone needed to turn around before the summit, it would be me. I dutifully filled my role as the grunt, and at the end of the climb, Peter asked me to share a beer with him and chat. Ed generously tipped me from his share of the client tips and then headed home, so it left some space for casual banter between Peter and me.

"You did amazing, Melis. It was awesome having you up there. I want you with me on every climb." I nodded as Peter laid down these little treats of praise for me to nibble on, grateful that I had been noticed in the right ways. "You are going to do big things. Who knows, you might even do more than me." He clinked his glass on mine with this suggestion, and gave a little smile. I could be good. I could be as good as him. I could be even better.

Peter was the big boss at RMI, and that title demanded a level of automatic reverence from all the guides. But Peter was also joked about regularly. He carried old, oval-shaped carabiners on his harness, a clear sign of his aging climbing knowledge. He never rock-climbed, or ice-climbed, and rarely even did any mountaineering outside of guiding. He didn't seem to love the mountains as much as he loved the spotlight. He hosted an adventure show on an obscure channel. One year, he filmed on Everest for the Discovery Channel. He was a good host; it was a natural extension of the charisma and charm he brought to guiding. That, combined with his good looks, straight teeth, and perfect hair, earned him the nickname Hollywood, mostly said behind his back. The guides joked about his old-school climbing, but when Hollywood came around, they clamored to share the spotlight for a moment. He moved easily, opportunities dangling from his long limbs.

I noted how Peter was clever and quick and smooth in almost every situation. He always said the right thing, whether it was completely true or not. He knew just how to position himself for the next step, and I envied his ability to move up continuously. I smiled at him and showered him with praise at every chance. I helped him look good in front of the clients, and he rewarded me by keeping me close. I would be his protégé. He would mold me into a guide as good and famous as him. I thought about my childhood dog, Mel, a wild animal who willingly stayed within his fence even though he knew how to escape. I thought of my dad, who existed in much the same way. Somehow, what they got seemed to outweigh what they lost. That was the equation of consenting captivity, and I willingly became captive, having practiced it for my entire life.

* * *

The summer of 2007 was like no other I had seen in my three years of guiding on Rainier. The mountain was melting and refreezing itself in revolt against the humans who wished to climb her flanks. It started with an abnormally low snowpack and continued to get worse with glaciers that were so actively rearranging themselves that a route would only stay climbable for two or three days at a time before it had to be rerouted entirely. The lack of snow made it harder to navigate those crevasses and made the route far more icy and challenging. It was August, and my own season was ending. I was thankful for that, as the burnout of climbing in highly stressful conditions was weighing me down. I wanted a break. I needed a break.

RMI had unofficially changed its policy regarding what happened when clients turned around before summiting—we no longer would have a single guide alone high on the mountain with more than two clients because of the need for technical ropework over the rock-hard blue ice, a type we refer to as "bulletproof." Quietly, as a kind of insurance, guides were axing marginal clients from climbing at rates like never before. If you weren't surefooted, fit, and adept at following directions, you wouldn't leave Camp Muir, the starting point of the technical climbing and the end of the approach hike. That was just the way it had to be to ensure the safety of both the guides and the clients.

Of course, it seemed to me that these rules didn't apply to Peter and the teams he was leading. No rules seemed to. He was the owner of the company. And for my last climb of the season, I would be his assistant.[*] We were guiding a media group put together by *Men's Journal.* The team included two writers, a Patagonia employee, a marketing executive from Mountain Hardwear, the brand-new CEO of Eddie Bauer, and the ad salesman, Gary, who had put the whole thing together. All the clients had some experience, but Mount Rainier didn't care, especially not this season.

We tried to thin out the group, putting them through the trials and challenges that would reveal signs of weakness. But thinning out wasn't happening—the clients all held tough when we increased the pace up to Camp Muir. They all followed the intricate instructions for how to self-arrest while sliding headfirst downhill on your back. When it came time to leave Muir, it was still all six of them, setting us up for huge

---

[*] Which really meant, again, doing all the work, leading the climb, and then stepping aside to let him receive the praise from the clients.

challenges ahead. We didn't have enough guides to maintain the ratio if some of them ran into trouble and had to retreat. There were other guides guiding other clients alongside us, which offered some comfort in these challenging conditions, but it was still risky. The night before we left Camp Muir, Peter circled all the guides to chat about strategy. It was going to be windy. The route was in horrible condition, icier than ever. There was no room for error.

The first few hours of the climb passed like the climbs before, with all the rope teams leaving Camp Muir together in a long string of bobbing headlamps in the night. Two or three climbers and one guide walked across the glacier, spread twenty-five feet apart and all attached to the same rope for safety. Each team stayed close to the one in front in a tight horizontal line so all the guides could assist one another as needed. We were still in the safe zone, a thousand feet below the area where the route suddenly turned from beginner to advanced. The guides moved at a brisk pace, trying once again to lose the clients who were anything less than perfect. This worked as planned, and at the first break, two guides turned around with four clients. At the next break, another two guides turned around with another four clients. That left Peter and two of the climbers on his rope and all three of my climbers remaining. Two guides, five climbers. We gave them a pep talk and attempted to fill them with fear: *You cannot continue from this point unless you know you can get to the summit and back down.* The icy flanks of the upper mountain stretched out in front of us as the sun cracked the horizon and the wind picked up. They all nodded their naïve reassurance. They could do it. They all promised they could.

Within the first twenty minutes of climbing out on the steep and firm ice, the rope behind me began to tighten. It was the one woman, the marketing executive. She was slowing down and tugging on the rope. "You have to keep up!" I yelled back to her. "You cannot pull on me here. It is too dangerous." She draped her body forward over her ice axe in the universal sign of exhaustion that all clients seemed to learn without ever being told. "I am dizzy," she whimpered up to me. I coiled in the rope as I keyed my radio. "Peter, it's Melissa. Trixie* is having issues. Can you hold there for a minute while I figure out what is going on?"

"Yep, no problem. I will regroup with my team as well."

As she came closer, I noticed the telltale lack of coordination that comes with true altitude sickness. Her description of feeling dizzy and nauseous, like she was floating away, confirmed my fear. She wasn't going to be climbing any farther. She needed to go down. Which meant, by the new rules, that Peter and all four other clients would need to go down as well. I asked her if she could climb short-roped close to me, another five minutes uphill, to meet with Peter's rope team. She agreed to try, and as I neared his rope, I keyed the radio again.

"Trixie needs to go down."

"Okay. I've got Ben, who needs to go down as well. He is getting sloppy." The relief washed away my nervousness as Peter said this. It wasn't going to be only my rope team who turned us around. Some days weren't meant for climbing, and I had no problem with that at all. As I approached the flat spot where Peter's team rested together, I noticed that Ben was not clipped into the rope, which was normal at a break where a client was preparing to turn around and head back to camp with a guide. Peter motioned me over for a private chat. "You will take Ben and Trixie down." He paused as I recoiled with surprise. That wasn't what I expected. This wasn't the plan. "You can also take Gary from my rope. He's good, he's very strong." I would go down, he said, and he would continue up with the Eddie Bauer CEO and the journalist. "The rest of my team is moving well and we will be fast. I bet we'll even catch you on the way down." His tone told me this wasn't a question; it was what I was going to do.

I shook my head as rage rose within me. He was sending me down with a client as backup. Even a strong client was still not a guide. This meant that I would be crossing hazardous terrain with three clients and,

---

* I have no idea what her name was, but it wasn't Trixie.

further, it meant Peter would be alone on the upper mountain with two. We would both be pushing outside of the safety plan that I thought the route required. I felt betrayed.

I looked Peter in the eyes. "This is not what we agreed to." We had been working closely together for three seasons, and I was comfortable enough to be firm with him. He had listened to me as I navigated one of my many breakups with Brad, assuring me that I was well enough established as a guide in my own right, and that any estrangement from my guide boyfriend wouldn't impact my job. We had filmed how-to videos together for his gear shop and shared bottles of wine, as friends.

The comfort I had with him was what allowed the space for my anger. He wasn't just a supervisor telling me what to do. He was Hollywood, and I knew him well. I felt like he cared far more about his businesses and his own fame than he did about the art of guiding. I also knew that just before the climb started, he had begun detailed negotiations with one of the clients, Neil, the new CEO of Eddie Bauer, to sponsor RMI and work closely with him. So, really, it shouldn't have come as a surprise that he would be willing to change the plan. Maybe he felt confident that the risk was low, or maybe he thought that his years of experience allowed him to make these sorts of game-time calls. I was angry that he made the decision despite my strong objection. At the time, I was cursing myself for ever thinking that what he cared about most somehow included me.

The route traversed 35-degree slopes, but the firm and glistening ice made every step critical. One wrong move and you could wind up sliding into oblivion. I put Gary on the front of the rope, tasking him with seeing the nonexistent path through the bulletproof ice and clipping into each of the fifteen anchor points we had created on our climb up. Stretched twenty-five feet behind him on the same rope was Ben, tired but still attentive enough to follow Gary. And another twenty-five feet would lead to Trixie, who I kept a few feet away from me on a shortened rope interval, a way to control clients who have unsure foot placement and protect the whole rope team from slipping into a tangled mess if someone falls. We began slowly snaking our way down, the sun now high above us but the wind increasing to a persistent growl. Gary clipped the anchors, known as a running belay, as he saw them and only meandered off the trail a few times, quickly correcting himself. Trixie was slow but getting better with each step of our descent.

My eyes were trained on Gary as he strolled right past the next anchor without clipping into it. "Gary! You missed the clip!" I yelled over the howl of the wind. The anchors were spread intentionally apart from one another to allow the rope team to stay attached to at least one at all times, and his missing it meant we had no anchors at all. We were just standing on the steep slopes, tethered only to one another.

As Gary turned to look uphill and reorient himself, Trixie crashed to her knees with incredible speed and force. The slope was steep enough and the rope between us short enough that her sudden move flipped me directly over her head in a sort of Hulk Hogan WWE wrestling move. And with that momentum, I started sliding at full speed down the icy slope, dragging Trixie behind me and quickly plucking both Ben and Gary off their feet to create a high-speed tangle of humans accelerating over ice and headed for the abyss of open crevasses below us. The surface was smooth minus a few cracks of ice, and this allowed us to quickly pick up incredible speed. My mind struggled to orient itself to which direction was even up. The guys, who were heavier, swung below Trixie and me in a nightmarish luge down the mountain. We were unstoppable. The solid ice wouldn't allow for any of us to self-arrest, and I knew it. This was how I was going to die.

And just as that thought settled across my brain, a sharp pain shot up my leg and my entire body vibrated to a screeching and sudden halt.

I was upside down, half-lodged by the leg in a crack of ice, and the three clients were sprawled on the rope below me. Adrenaline flooded my body as the fear hit me. I quickly placed an ice screw and clipped our rope into it. An anchor. We had an anchor. We weren't going to slide to our deaths. We had stopped after a short but high-speed fall, and the crevasses that would swallow us up were still far below. What felt like an eternity of sliding toward death had been only a few seconds of uncontrolled slipping. We had gotten very lucky.

I yelled to the clients individually, asking if they were hurt. They all replied that they were okay, and I brought them safely toward me, anchored by an ice screw and the rope. My leg throbbed just below my knee where it was jammed in the ice, but I could move and put weight on it, and I wasn't bleeding, so I moved on quickly to taking care of the clients. The slope where we had come to a stop wasn't as steep, but it was still icy. Once I got them all close to me and anchored, I assessed them, discovering that, by some miraculous fate, they were all completely fine. Except Gary. He desperately needed a blue bag. I distanced him slightly to shit in a bag.* Everyone seemed shockingly unaware of the brush with death we had just experienced.

My leg throbbed, but I wanted off the mountain. I called down to Camp Muir on the radio and let them know my rope team had taken a fall, but we were okay, and moving again. We limped our way back into the camp while Peter went to the summit and began making his way down. He didn't catch us like he said he would, and when he returned to camp, I had already been back for more than an hour.

More than an hour is plenty of time to let the adrenaline fade and the pain, physical and emotional, to rise. I was pissed. He had ignored his own rules and sacrificed me so he could get a CEO to the summit and secure a new sponsorship. He cared only about himself. Capital P, capital W. I didn't want to climb with him ever again. As Peter trotted back into camp wearing the pride of being the only team to summit that day, he came toward me. I was still shaken by the closest call I had ever had in the mountains. I felt the fragility of this life and our choices and a particular, blistering anger that I had almost died because of a choice someone else made for me. "Hey, Melis, how did that go? Sorry about that."

---

* He asked me out after the climb. That takes a special kind of person. I said yes and then stood him up at the airport, faking a kidney stone to account for ghosting him. That also takes a special kind of person.

Another guide stepped in. "I wouldn't talk to her right now." I looked up at Peter, my eyes narrowed and still, conveying all the things I would never be brave enough to say. I didn't want him to hear my anger or my fear. I didn't want him to see me as weak. I just wanted him to sit with his own decision-making, punctuated by my silence. I would tell him another day, though that day never came.* But I would not risk my life for his ego again. I was done. I wouldn't be as good as Peter; I would be better.

---

* Or, I guess that day is today.

8.

POSSIBILITIES

2007: Seattle, Washington

I walked briskly in the chilly and damp Seattle air on a November night. It felt like the beginning of a life I couldn't imagine myself in. I had said yes to attending a celebrity-filled L.A. party I knew little about, and also to guiding my first trip on Mount Everest, both with my client Mike. The world that had existed quietly alongside my own, never available to me, was going to become mine. I just had to find something to wear.

I'd met Mike on a Rainier climb the previous summer. He was a successful and fit middle-aged white man who had found reprieve from the corporate grind by challenging himself in the mountains. He was a typical client in nearly every way, except that he had already climbed the seven summits, including Everest in 2004 with Dave Morton as his guide. Our Rainier climb had turned into an eventful one when another client developed sudden blindness and we terminated the normal flow of the climb to help the client down safely. I led the rescue. Mike witnessed the events unfold, and after the climb, he asked me if I would consider going with him to Everest. He was planning to go back and said that he wanted a guide with rescue skills and leadership like I had shown that day.

I hesitated, unsure if he was serious. It was one of two questions that nearly every client on Rainier would ask—"Do you want to climb Everest?" and "Have you read *Into Thin Air*?" I played my role dutifully as a young mountain guide and said, "Yes! Of course!" to both questions, even though the true answer for both was no, at least superficially. Everest seemed like a shiny treat that my clients or Peter would dangle over me to see how high I would jump. Most of those clients would never actually get there themselves. I had refused to look too closely at Everest, certain that it might never be a place for me. I didn't know of any other guides in their early twenties who got a chance to go there, and certainly no women. Brad had been lucky enough to join his best friend and fellow mountain guide on a sponsored climb of Everest the past spring. We were in one of our temporary breakups when he left, and as I followed his climb from a distance, my desire to have what he had made me want to be close to him again. Deep under that truth of not wanting to climb Everest was another truth: I didn't want to simply climb Everest, I wanted to *guide* Everest. I wanted what the people in power had. But girls didn't guide on Everest, so why climb it at all? My ego told me I certainly didn't need to read Jon Krakauer's book to know the story; clients regularly recited their favorite parts to me, which always included the women in peril or, worse, as the cause of the tragedy, with the men as the heroes.

It wasn't until October that I had the courage to email Mike and ask if he was still thinking of returning to Everest. Brad and I had briefly gotten back together in the summer, but the jealousy and fighting started again by August, and when he left for another Himalayan expedition, we broke up again. My season had ended tumultuously in every way, and my relationship with Peter was also strained after our final climb. I had started to seriously question if I should keep working for Peter on Rainier. But I knew enough not to decide to quit right then; by spring I would likely forget the flaws in guiding for Peter and be eager to head back. At the end of the season, Peter had dangled an offer: Sign on to a five-year sponsorship with Eddie Bauer and help him and a small team reinvigorate the outdoor brand with true technical outerwear. It was the reward he had secured for guiding the CEO to the summit on our climb, and now he was offering to share it with me. I was suspicious of these promises because I was suspicious of him. I thought maybe it was time to ascend without Peter's help. Maybe Mike's invitation to Everest had come at the perfect time.

Mike was in the process of finalizing his team. He was going to climb with Alpine Ascents,* one of RMI's competitors, and yes, he still wanted me to join. He asked me to meet him for dinner in downtown Seattle at a swanky Fourth Avenue wine bar to discuss his vision for the climb. The notion of meeting him for a meal at such a nice place gave me the oddly familiar feeling of being Julia Roberts in *Pretty Woman*. I shook off that thought and booked a room for sixty-seven bucks a night at the Best Western Loyal Inn ten blocks away. I put on my cleanest jeans[†] and my "fancy" cowboy boots and walked into the dimly lit otherworld of an upscale Seattle wine bar. Mike saw me and stood, then leaned in to hug me.[‡]

He was soft-spoken yet exuberant, slightly nerdy but funny, with a quick sense of humor. As the VP at one of the big tech companies, he existed in a world of dinners and drinks with people like Bono and Mitt Romney.[§] It seemed to me that he cared about the world and was driven to see a change in the inequities that bothered him the most. Through his work, he had become aware of Product (RED), a business model

---

* A guide service with an owner who periodically tried to lure me over to working for them because experienced female guides were a commodity.

† But still dirty.

‡ His jeans were actually quite clean.

§ Not at the same time. Though I would want to be at that dinner.

started by Bono and Bobbi Shriver, brother of the former California first lady Maria Shriver and a Kennedy cousin. They were teaching businesses how to leverage the desire of consumers to do good by creating products that were uniquely branded; the companies would donate some of the profits to the global fund and to fighting the worldwide AIDS crisis, especially in Africa. Mike had recently gone to a clinic in Ghana and had seen firsthand how access to anti-retroviral drugs was changing people's lives. "When I was in Africa, I decided these stories needed to be told," he said earnestly, when explaining to me why he wanted to return to Everest. "We can climb in sixty days, and in that time, we can follow people who are receiving medication and share their stories of hope and what the work that Product (RED) is truly doing. It will be the most widely covered 'real time' Everest trip in history!" In sixty days, he said, we would see a mother become strong and well enough to care for her children. We would see a child begin to dream of a life and not only their death. And we, he told me, would use the billboard that is Everest paired with the media machine he knew to tell their stories.

Mike's passion piqued my curiosity. It wasn't totally clear to me why he wanted me there, though, and I had to know this before I could agree to climb with him.

"Why me?" I pressed him. "I mean, why not just climb with Dave Morton again?"

He gave a knowing little smirk and swirled his wine in the way that people who know how to handle wineglasses do. I noticed his perfectly manicured fingers delicately holding the stem of the glass, a contrast to my glass, now foggy with my dirty fingerprints because I was holding it like an ogre.

"Well, a few reasons. The first one is that you deserve a chance to go there. I can see that, and if I can give that to you, I want to. You can look into it; I have a long history of elevating competent women whenever I can." He paused here, looking me in the eye intensely and causing me to slightly squirm, unsure how I should react. "But mostly it is because of the rescue on Rainier. I realized how essential it was to have someone with rescue skills. And medical skills. I have never thought I needed it, so I didn't know what wasn't there. So, I want you there." This made me happy. I wanted to be valued for my skill set above all else. I wanted him to need me, not just want me. And I also wondered if he was smart enough to know this and if that was why he added that part.

"Yes. Okay. I will do it. I am in!" I chirped enthusiastically, trying to convey my excitement. Inside, I felt the swirl of possibilities mingle with my fear that something would take this chance away from me. Could this really be happening? Could I really pull this off, and have a chance to climb the highest mountain on Earth? I felt my cheeks flush as the swell of adrenaline pulsed through my body. He reached across the hightop table and grabbed my hands in his own, giving them a little squeeze. "It is going to be great. Okay, next question. What are you doing Thursday?" he asked me, while still holding my hands in his. What was I doing? I couldn't say that I had nothing going on, which was the truth. I was homeless by choice, living in the back of my truck again. I didn't have any guiding work for at least another month, and I wasn't scheduled to teach any medical courses between now and then.

Mike continued in my silence. "Friday is World AIDS Day, and Bobbi and Bono are throwing a party Thursday night in Santa Monica. I am going and announcing our Product (RED) climb there. And it would be great if *my* guide could join me. I will take care of the flight and everything. You could be home by Friday afternoon." I swallowed and fell deeper into my *Pretty Woman* story. He was plucking me off the street and dressing me in fancy clothes and asking me to join him in his world, far from my own. Mike had all the power to elevate my career and standing in the community of guides and climbers. All I had to do was say yes. I could choose what I said yes to, right? I could say no if he asked for too much in return, right? I assured myself that though he had the power now, I still had a choice. Inside, I hushed the voice that questioned whether his admiring looks were for my skills or my body.

I was so excited to think that this fantasy of life he was offering me—and all the opportunity it contained—was actually happening! I would borrow some heels. I had a little black dress. I was going to do this, and the slurry of fear and excitement turned electric inside me, the buzz muting out the sheer unlikeliness of it all. I sipped my wine, said goodbye, and ended the night tucked safely into my Best Western room while Mike drove away in his little custom Porsche, our lives diverging once again from the faux commonality we shared over drinks. He didn't look nearly as comfortable in a down suit as he did in a business suit. And in the city, we reversed roles, as I pretended to know that the engine of the Porsche is in the trunk.

* * *

When I arrived in Los Angeles on Thursday, a fancy black car took me from the airport to the Four Seasons in Beverly Hills, where a basket of fruit awaited my arrival in my room, or I should say *our* room. Mike told me he would sleep on the sofa bed and I could take the bedroom. He was going to run some errands while I showered and got ready. I unfolded my clothes onto the pristine white bedsheets and jumped in the shower, lathering myself with a soap I hoped could wash away my life up until then and lather me in a new world of opulence and luxury. I smelled the aroma of belonging. It was intoxicating.

As I got out of the shower and swaddled myself in the fluffy white robe that came with the room, Mike knocked on the bedroom door.* I cracked it open, showing just the towel on my head and robe. "Sorry," he said shyly. "I just wanted to let you know we will leave here at five." His words came out muffled as he looked down at the floor, as though I weren't wearing an oversize robe. He looked at me as though I was wearing nothing, both curious and embarrassed.

---

* A hotel room with a whole separate room to sleep in, connected to the living area, was quite the upgrade from the shitty Best Western in Seattle.

"No, it's okay," I said, trying to put him at ease. "I was going to ask you . . . I don't have many choices, but what should I wear? I mean, is it fancy?"

"As is. What you were wearing today is great." I nodded, and he left. I had been wearing the same pair of nine-dollar summer-sale Old Navy jeans I had on at the wine bar on Monday. My nice cowboy boots made me seem at least two inches taller. I'd bought them with a gift card a client had given me as a tip the previous summer. And I was wearing a Product (RED) T-shirt from the Gap, which Mike had bought me while we wandered around Rodeo Drive that afternoon. It said "INSPI(RED)" on it. That was going to be our team, he told me, Team Inspired. I brushed my hair, applied mascara, and tried to project all the confidence I was lacking. On the snow and ice, I knew I had value. I kept people safe and alive and pushed them to push themselves. But thrust into a dinner party with wealthy and famous people, I felt like the girl who was raised in a silver trailer. I felt overly simple and homely. So I stood taller, breathed a little deeper, and told myself I could do anything. I could do this.

I tried to get my bearings as we arrived at the gated mansion. There was the ocean. There was the sky. The December air seemed deceptively warm, but this was California, so maybe it was always warm. I didn't need my dirt-stained Patagonia jacket, but it felt weird to leave it behind. It was a status symbol and part of my identity in my real life, but it felt out of place and useless here. Mike was wearing slacks and a fancy T-shirt covered by a blazer. He looked cool, somehow formal and casual at the same time. I writhed in my skin, wondering how out of place I was going to be.

My answer came quickly as we were greeted by a trio of women in full-length evening gowns. One was deep red and backless, adorned with shimmers that made its wearer look like a firefly as she moved in the dimly lit entryway. Another was white and resembled a wedding dress, with layers of sheer material. The women were beautiful and perfectly put together, with hair and nails and makeup and shoes that made me uncomfortably aware of all my own informal parts. I smiled and stepped out of their way. Maybe they were going somewhere else after this. That thought crashed to the floor as we entered a room of formally clad adults in black-tie dress and beautiful jewels. I felt like someone's child. Or someone's intern. Or worse, just a prop.

"Do you want to check your coat?" a man asked me. He looked more like me. He was a worker. I was a worker. I wanted to ask him if I could just help him with the coat check. But instead, I reluctantly gave him my Patagonia jacket in exchange for a little paper ticket. I had no idea what to do with the ticket because I had never checked a coat before, and certainly never at someone's home. But then, this was unlike any home I had ever seen.

Mike ushered me around the estate through a series of large rooms that flowed into a giant backyard enclosed with an event tent set with gorgeous tables. Flowers and candles and lights were placed perfectly, as if it were a long-planned wedding reception. Mike navigated the rooms, introducing me to people who struggled not to look me up and down. I felt the tension in the conversation, the pause of people wanting to ask me what I was doing there. As we stood at the bar waiting for a glass of wine, Mike joked with a professional woman he knew. "What do you think her job is?" He nodded his chin at me as I darted a glance back at him. "I will give you three choices. She is the new head of marketing for Ann Taylor, she is a mountain guide who climbs Everest, or she is a math professor at Berkeley." He smirked at his cleverness as the woman smiled and turned her head to the side, looking me up and down with a patronizing giggle.

"You have to give me at least one realistic option! I am guessing she's an actor, so all of them!"

My insides clenched. I couldn't tell if I was a joke or if Mike was just so proud of how incredulous it was that he had found this young blond girl who was going to guide him up Everest. I stood steady in my boots. I tried not to shrink but to grow. Don't hide. Be noticed. Be confident.

Just then, Bobbi Shriver came rushing toward us. He was tall and tan, with the chiseled face of someone who belongs on TV. His suit was perfectly tailored and looked both formal and comfortable. The contrast mirrored his movements, which felt both smooth and chaotic. His brown hair looked intentionally messy in that cool California way. "This! Look, everyone!" he shouted above the casual din of conversation as he swept in and placed his arm around me, his drink resting on my shoulder. "This is the best-dressed woman here!" He pointed to my Product (RED) shirt. I wanted to disappear. I still couldn't tell if I was the butt of a joke, but I was sure he couldn't be serious.

Instead, I smiled and looked down as all the eyes around us fell on me. "Just trying to be supportive," I whispered, mostly to him.

Mike jumped to my rescue quickly. "She is a mountain guide!" he exclaimed, as though the words were a foreign language to the audience surrounding us. "She is homeless and just travels the world to climb, and next spring she will be *my* guide on Everest!"

Homeless. I wished he hadn't said that. Homelessness meant something different in L.A. than it did in the mountain guide community, with our often nomadic lives. And I hadn't climbed Everest yet, so I couldn't answer a single question about it. I tried to explain to Bobbi that being homeless was a choice so I could travel to climb, but he seemed to struggle to understand me. "You could live in my pool house if you want!" he said, loudly laughing. Then he pranced off to the next easy exchange, leaving me in my discomfort.

I said to myself, *You can do anything for an hour,* again and again, like a mantra. Mike ushered me around and made sure my wineglass stayed full. I was thankful for him and unsure of him at the same time. Who did he think I was? Maybe I looked different to him in the mountains and now, seeing me here, he would realize his mistake. I didn't belong in the big leagues. I didn't belong with him.

The night ended far later than I hoped it would. I searched my pockets for the little paper with the numbers on it that would prove my identity. I couldn't find it anywhere. I panicked as we approached the coat check. "I can't find my ticket," I said, ashamed, to the man at the counter.

He looked at me and paused for a moment. "Don't worry, honey. I know which one is yours." I scrunched my nose, unsure if that was a compliment or an insult or just a perfect summary of my whole night.

I folded my jacket under my arm and swung the heavy front door open to see Mike, already in the car. "That was so great!" he said as I climbed in. "Thank you!" We exchanged little stories about various encounters in our night on the drive back to the hotel. I entered the room that I didn't belong in and kicked my boots off. I threw the brand-new Gap T-shirt on the chair and pulled my comfy tank-top over my head. I wanted my skin back. I wanted to feel like myself. I was in one of the most comfortable and luxurious hotels in the world, but I yearned for the sleeping bag in the back of my old pickup. Mike kept his word and retreated to the couch, though I felt the heavy expectation in the room that if I told him he could come to my bed, he would have. I grabbed the remote and crawled into the fluffy, extravagant bed. *Kung Fu Panda* was on TV, featuring a clumsy misfit panda who dreams of becoming a kung fu legend. *I can do this,* I thought. If the panda can do it, I can too. I can be the Kung Fu Panda.

My breath was caught in my chest as I lay there watching the movie. Was I getting myself into something I wouldn't be able to get out of? Mike had promised to bring me to Everest, but none of the details had yet been worked out. Who would I work for? What would he pay me? What would be expected of me? I felt like the night of opulence had been a tease, him showing me what my life could be like if I stayed close to him. It was subtle but familiar: a man with power offering me freedom from my current life and access to his. I thought about Officer Jones sitting across the table from me, telling me how good my life was going to be if I just left with him. I thought about Peter, offering me sponsorship if I just stayed close to him. I thought about the gaze of these men and how artfully they danced around the suggestion that I was an object of their attention for anything other than professional intentions. But the hand on my leg, the holding of my lower back, the cheek kiss for a greeting turning into a lip kiss, all told me that what they were offering was going to cost me.

I wanted Mike to be different but I also wanted so badly to get to Everest and have a chance to change my own life. If I climbed to the summit, for my first time, at age twenty-four and as a guide . . . I was sure it would change everything and I would no longer have to engage in flirtations and touches and glances for power. The climb ahead of me, just to get to the mountain, would be far more difficult than the simple movement of crampons puncturing ice on the ascent of Everest. But if I could do it, maybe then I could be free.

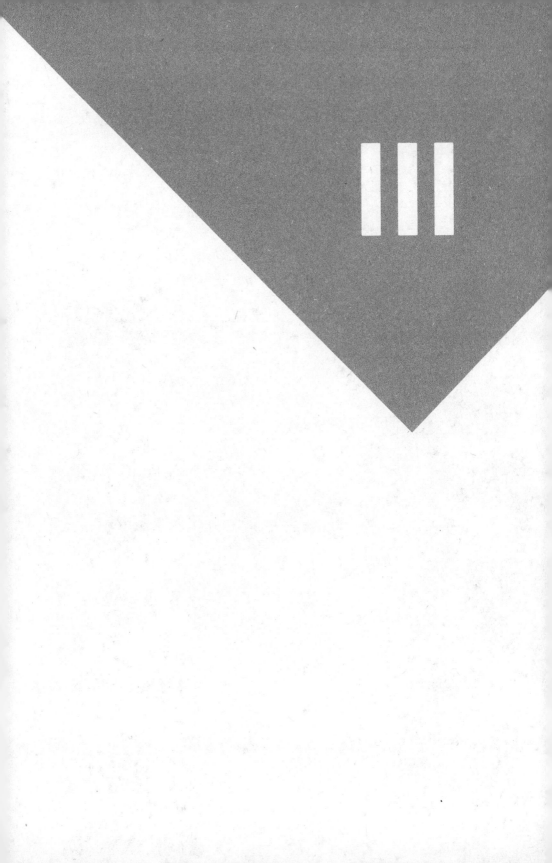

9.

A MAN'S WORLD

2008: Mount Everest, Nepal

The old Twin Otter jerked to a stop on the uphill runway situated at 9,000 feet. I could see out the windshield, and directly in front of us was a grassy hillside, and behind that, a giant stone mountain. Red, blue, and green roofs topped tiny stone buildings that lined the runway. This was the entrance to Everest and the final point of motorized travel. From here, it was all walking on the dusty and well-traveled trails for thirty-five miles into Everest Base Camp.

As we got off the plane, the cold mountain air hit my face as my neck craned to try to see the tops of the peaks that surrounded us. It was stunning. The sun was sprinkling the snowcapped peaks with its rays, making them glitter and shine. These were the tallest mountains in the world. This was the path that was going to take me to climb them. The smell of wood smoke from the small houses hit my nose and mixed with the crisp cold of the mountain air, sending a shiver down my back. I never thought I would see this place with my own eyes, and now here I was.

"What are you listening to?" Mike asked as we slowly moved our way up the hill toward Everest Base Camp. I handed him my headphones with their long, tangled cord tied in knots from being shoved into my pockets. Sharing with him the feminist acoustic poetry of Ani DiFranco that had been my main companion was a little embarrassing, but it was a welcome break from the way he insisted on pointing out every curve of the trail and notable peak in the distance. This shouldn't have bothered me. It was, after all, why I was here. This was my first time in Nepal, and on Everest. But not his, and he liked to make sure that I remembered that. The Mike who had shown me his opulent world of dinner parties and nice wine was not the Mike I was walking with. This Mike was out of his element, and that insecurity caused him to constantly remind me that he was why I was here. I might be a guide, but I was an assistant guide on my first trip to the Himalayas and he was the client and the reason I was here at all, and it felt like he reveled in each chance to remind me of my inexperience in this place compared to his.

I had been hesitant to agree to join the trip because of my lack of experience, but the logistics were quickly worked out so that I would be an apprentice of sorts, under the mentorship of Dave Morton, who had been on Everest for three seasons already. He had guided Mike on his first summit four years prior, and he had agreed to take me under his wing and show me how to work on a mountain this big.

The trail was as wide as two yaks and sprawled out for miles in front of us: dusty, dry, and the only way to get to Base Camp. It was a new place to me but had the familiarity of the trails I had tromped in the Colorado woods as a child. The trees were the same, and the brushy juniper reminded me of the cedar trees I would peel the bark from as a kid.

The journey was more than thirty miles from where we started walking, and in that distance, we would ascend over nine thousand more feet, up and down and up again, until we reached our temporary home at the base of the Khumbu icefall on the south side of Everest. I didn't know much about the Khumbu icefall, except that it was distinctly marked on a map that came out of a National Geographic special on Everest and the name "Khumbu" got stuck in my head for days after I saw it the first time. *KOO-m-BOO. Koommmmbooo. Koomboo.* The word was symmetrical and had a peaceful rhythm in my mouth—nothing at all like the actual place, a dangerous and chaotic flow of avalanching ice that could kill you with its unpredictability.

The first days of the trek toward the icefall had been much busier than I expected. But then again, I hadn't known what to expect. I had been avoiding all things Everest since I started climbing, sure that I would never see it myself. I hadn't wanted to learn about a place that I would never be able to go, and so the busy trail surprised me nearly as much as everyone's apprehension about the flight in. I hadn't read much about that either. If I had, I would have learned that the broken four hundred yards of pavement that angled steeply uphill and ended in a brick wall embedded in a hillside was considered one of the most dangerous runways in the world. And we would land on it in the old twin propeller plane. I was glad I didn't know this as we boarded the plane with twelve other nervous people and I noticed that the airplane's tires were particularly bare and worn bald on the outer edges. The flight went without a hitch, but when we landed everyone clapped.

The tiny village that housed the runway, called Lukla (*Lou-kla*), is the gateway to the high Himalayan peaks. It was there that I became acquainted with teahouses and the generous and kind Sherpas who owned them. The simple buildings were built for tourists, with benches bordering the main rooms and little intricately carved wooden tables in front of the benches for eating soup and drinking tea. The local tea is called dudchia (translated as "milk tea"), a sweet and creamy mixture of black tea, yak milk,* and heaps of sugar. I curved my hands around the

---

* Actually, nak milk. Naks are female yaks, and yaks don't make milk.

plastic teacups and appreciated the smell of juniper burning in the little potbelly stove in the center of the room. It reminded me of the smell of my childhood and the woodstove in the little silver trailer.*

This first teahouse in Lukla served as an orientation to Sherpa culture and what the next two weeks would be like, as we hiked our way toward our camp at 17,800 feet. Being in a room surrounded by people who didn't look like me reminded me of going to school on the Southern Ute Indian reservation. The Sherpa women, adorned with turquoise and coral, reminded me of the tribal members with kind eyes, few words, and clear power. It was a subtle but significant matriarchy. I learned that you never eat or shake with your left hand, as it is the one reserved for wiping after you do your business in the bathroom. I learned that *namaste* means "hello" in Nepali, but *tashi delek* (pronounced "tashi delay") is the proper greeting in Sherpa.

Dave was mostly kept busy with the larger group of clients that were traveling adjacent to us, so this left Mike as my expert location guru. "Look! That peak is sacred. Unclimbed but beautiful!" He pointed out the first peak we could see and told me it was called Khumbi-La as he thrust hand sanitizer my way. "Cover your face with your neck gaiter!" he scolded. "You will get the Khumbu-cough."† Mike clearly enjoyed sharing his insights, and though I felt slightly like his child, I tried to dutifully obey. Down low, I figured, he could act like the guide. I tried to take in his shared knowledge with humility, though that had never been my strong suit. I wanted space and quiet to observe as much as I could and soak it all in. But I was here for Mike, and if he wanted to teach me all the ways of being a guest here, I wasn't going to bristle at that.‡

---

* Sherpa families burn juniper regularly as a form of offering and prayer, and it is the pervasive smell in the valley.

† The area was well known for causing a dry and persistent cough from the dust, dry air, and high elevation.

‡ But really, I did bristle at it. And I like to imagine I hid my disdain for being treated

We hiked for hours, weaving in and out of other tourists, mostly trekkers but some climbers. It was a game of sizing everyone up. Did that person look like a climber? Would they make it to the summit? Had they been here before? I quickly learned that you didn't need to wonder for long who was a climber. They would tell you. And if they had been there before, they would definitely tell you that. Mike did it in a way I think he viewed as subtle. "When I summited Everest in 2004 . . ." prefaced most of his observations. Occasionally he would drop a fact about the temperature or wind on summit day, just in case anyone was still unaware that he had been there before.

After the first few hours of ups and downs through a sprinkle of tiny villages, the groups started to spread out, allowing the trek to feel majestic and wild. As we climbed the switchbacks toward a rushing river—one that poured from the Khumbu icefall—I began to feel the smallness that nature has always bestowed upon me graciously. The river was wilder than I would ever be. The mountains were rebellious and independent, shooting to impossible heights and grazing the stars. And I was just a person, down here, on a dusty trail, trying to take it all in curiously on my soul journey.

After the first days of travel, our movements became predictable and rhythmic. We would wake at six a.m. with the sunrise and drink hot dudchia and coffee in the cold dining room. We would pack our duffels with sleeping bags and books and the porters would come and sling them over their backs, traipsing off as though they were carrying only feathers and not fifty pounds of creature comforts. We ate boiled eggs and flatbreads called chapati and then started hiking toward our next village.

The days lasted for four or five hours as we ascended one or two thousand feet to a new village with an identical teahouse. We would

---

like a child, but I have been in my body long enough now to know that I likely gave him a look that spilled my contempt for not only his teaching me, but the patriarchy in general.

drink from our teacups and play cards before dinner and then eat and retire to our sleeping bags to repeat the sequence the next day. It might have been boring if it weren't for the dramatic and ever-changing land-scape and weighty anticipation of where we were heading. Peaks formed pinnacles and shot straight up into the sky, adorned by jewels of ice that seemed to stay on the steep flanks by magic alone. My neck and heart felt sore each night from gazing up at giants I never thought I would have the chance to see. I wrote in my journal but felt afraid to even write the words that I was here, approaching Everest, fearful that if I spoke it out loud it would all go away.

That fear didn't come from nowhere. Just a few weeks before we were set to depart the U.S. for Nepal, Mike called to tell me that the Everest season was being canceled. China was hosting the Olympics that year and they wanted to carry a torch to the summit from the Chi-nese side. This, embarrassingly, was the first time I realized that Everest was both in China (or Tibet more specifically) and Nepal. But my geo-graphic ignorance was the least of it: Everest was going to be canceled. The Chinese apparently were fearful that climbers from Nepal could protest to free Tibet and possibly be seen from the north side, so they requested that Nepal close climbing. Nepal was apt to do what China wanted them to in the ever-unfair power dynamic of a tiny developing country bordered by a big and powerful neighbor. "Let's keep our tick-ets and go anyway," said Mike. "If we just trek, we just trek. Who knows, things could change." He was hopeful but I felt heartbroken. This whole thing had seemed too good to be true, so it probably was. But I was still excited for a twenty-four-hour flight across the world, so I wouldn't be the one to say no. Like most of this journey so far, I was along for the ride.

After we arrived, the restrictions slowly let up and we were allowed to ascend with various checkpoints and threats that our permits would be revoked. The main restriction that stayed in place was that we wouldn't be allowed to travel above Camp Two until the Chinese team had made it to the summit. This wasn't insignificant. The restriction would hamper our acclimatization by keeping us at 22,000 feet and not allowing our bodies to adjust to the higher camps before the weather changed and the summit push had to begin. But everyone agreed it was a risk that we could take to have a chance at all.

Even as the tallest mountain in the world, Everest remained hidden, tucked behind a whole range of peaks that protected her from our view. Each day of the approach toward Base Camp we inched closer and closer to seeing her, until one day we turned a corner and there she was. Jomolangma, as the Sherpas called her.* Her neck and crown poked above all the peaks that surrounded her, a dark black pyramid perched in the sky. The rock looked like it had white spiderwebs draped over it, decorating the peak and making it both amazing and spooky and different from any other mountain I had seen. The thin air was no match for how her presence could take your breath away. But just as we got our first glimpse of her, she dipped back behind the peaks in the foreground. It seemed beautiful to me that to climb Everest meant that you wouldn't see the summit again until the summit day. You would have to toil and work diligently toward something you just had to believe was out there. No peeking. And so, my view turned down and back to the dusty trail, tromped smooth by the sometimes-bare feet of porters, the soft hooves of the yaks, and the expensive trekking shoes of the tourists. I put in my headphones and daydreamed my way up the trail, always in sight of Mike. Sometimes he got ahead of me and sometimes he stayed behind. Sometimes we talked but often I slid an earbud in and we moved together in silence.

"You're singing?" he asked as he trekked up beside me, catching me off-guard.

"No," I said, shaking my head. "Or maybe. I'm just listening to Ani

---

* Some say "Jomolangma," while other Sherpas say "Chomolungma," and others even say "Chamulongmu," as the written words have evolved alongside the regional dialects.

DiFranco. I think this is my favorite song. She just says what I wish I could say."

I felt exposed, but there was really no way out. I handed him my headphones and turned the dial on my iPod back to start the song over.

I have to act just as strong as I can
Just to preserve a place where I can be who I am

That sentence described the years that had led me here. It was an act of preservation. So many of my actions were.

When Mike was finished listening, he handed me back my headphones. "All men aren't the same," he said, with a slight emotional crack in his words, as though he might cry. I knew that he needed to feel like he wasn't one of *them,* and for that to work I needed to tell him he was different.

"Of course, *you* aren't that way," I said, swallowing hard, acting just as strong as I could, preserving that little place that would allow me to survive over the next two months. I wondered if he knew that I knew he had the power.

Brad was also on Everest that spring season, guiding a different client on a different team. We were back together in the ever-tentative dance of our relationship, and having him close but at a distance actually felt like a gift. It was a small familiar comfort in this very foreign (to me) experience. We were on our own journeys, and he didn't own mine. And our chances to meet up were rare; I had no idea how big Everest Base Camp was until I got there and realized that his camp was a forty-five-minute walk from mine. We could rarely align our schedules to see each other, which was fine with me.

The weeks ticked by as I learned the ins and outs of climbing and guiding the highest peak in the world. Mike may have played the tour guide when we were trekking, but when it came time to step a crampon on the glacier, he would fall silent and subservient to my skills and experience. The familiar crunch of my crampons piercing the glacier in the pre-dawn climbs became my new soundtrack. The work of climbing above 19,000 feet toward Camp Two was arduous even for the experienced, and I soaked in all of the challenge willingly. I watched how Dave moved and how he rested, and mimicked both. I drank water when he did and ate bowls of ramen by his side, hoping to absorb all his knowledge and experience. He had grown up in a family with two sisters, the younger sixteen years his junior and a couple years younger than me, so he fell easily into his big brother role. He would share his playlist with me but rib me for not knowing the Nirvana songs. He was patient and careful to include me as much as possible, even when I would annoy him with my endless questions. He wasn't moody at all, and that stability along with the gentle sharing of his knowledge made me feel a sense of belonging that often eluded me, even in the mountains. This was what I came here for. It was hard, but it was home.

Most of my previous years of climbing translated here, but there were a few things that only Everest could teach. I learned how to quickly descend fixed lines by wrapping them around my arm and facing my body downhill, running down the slope like Spider-Man. I learned how oxygen tanks worked and how the regulators could fail. I learned that Mike didn't like being the slowest one, and he didn't like being too hot or too cold. He did like telling the other clients his clothing suggestions for summit day. But since we weren't allowed above the 22,000-foot mark of Camp Two because of the Chinese restrictions, the summit seemed impossibly far away. Each day, we checked in on the progress of the Chinese team on the north side, hoping they would get to the summit early. In the meantime, we hung out in a dining tent at Camp Two, huddled together around metal folding tables to play cards and pass the time.

During one of those games, Brad made the journey from his camp to ours and peeked his head in the door. His space at Camp Two was closer, but still a solid twenty-minute walk uphill, so I was surprised to see him. But I tried to stand and scoot my way past the other three guys in the card game (Mike; a Mexican climber, Davide; and a Sherpa,

Dawa) to greet him. "You made it up here!" I smiled as I tried to unzip the door fully and allow him in.

"I just came to say hi. But I'm going." He looked at me with an empty expression that I knew well: I was in trouble.

"Wait, I can come talk to you," I said.

He had already turned to leave. "Don't bother." His words were a near whisper, his back to me as he walked away.

I stood at the door, my body still half inside the tent, and debated what to do. He was mad, and, from most of our past fights, I could guess that it was because I was surrounded by men who weren't him. I didn't have the energy to fight with him here. I let him go. I went back to the cards and resigned myself to face the consequences of that choice.

Later that day when I bundled up and put on my boots to journey to his camp, he met me at his personal tent by opening the zipper no more than a face-size gap. "Don't come in here." He said it without emotion, which wasn't good. I had learned from the storms of my mother that no emotion was far more dangerous than anger.

"What did I *do*?" I asked, genuinely curious.

"We just shouldn't be together. It is clear that you want attention more than you want to be with me, so go." His voice was rising now. "Go! Go get it!" He zipped the door shut.

Did he just break up with me? I thought to myself. *Here? On Everest at Camp Two?* It felt as ridiculous as it was, and as I walked back to my camp I tried to compartmentalize the situation, saving my energy for the climb ahead. I would have to deal with this, and him, later. But that night I couldn't sleep. The on-again, off-again nature of Brad's moods and our relationship had worn me down, and I was mad at him for trying to control my summit attempt on Everest with the same bullshit he had been doing for years. Whenever something good came my way, if it wasn't directly because of something he had done for me, he tried to ruin it. And he was doing it again. But I knew that I couldn't let him take this from me. I wasn't working with him or for him. I was separating myself. I was here to do this so that I could untether myself from him completely and get opportunities because of this new accomplishment and experience and not who my boyfriend was. Fuck him for trying to take that from me. I wouldn't let him.

* * *

My crampons felt secure as they crunched into the firm snow on the Khumbu glacier, low on the slopes of Everest. The air was dry and cold but the wind was mostly friendly. I found the climbing to be remarkably like the slopes of Rainier, just bigger and harder in the very thin air of the high altitudes. Everest's base camp was three thousand feet higher than the summit of Rainier; its summit was two Rainiers stacked on top of each other. The difference was palpable. Steeps felt steeper, and the slightest change in weather would feel far more extreme than the forecast indicated. A fifteen-mile-per-hour gust of wind could feel like nothing more than a stiff breeze on the flanks of Rainier, but on Everest, with temperatures so close to freezing, the slightest wind would freeze your face and fingers. But the language of crampons on the glacier, apparently, was a universal one.*

As we worked through the weeks of climbing needed to adjust to the altitude, we moved up the mountain, slept in camps perched in impossibly beautiful locations, and headed back down to rest at Base Camp. And then did the same thing again, hoping to be stronger. Much to my surprise, Base Camp was a social and buzzing international community. I hadn't been able to understand until we were there how much of climbing really big mountains was just resting at the base camp. There were more than thirty mountain guides, and I was the only woman. I quickly learned that women are a rarity on Everest, making up less than 10 percent of the population. I asked some of the veterans about this, but no

---

* I had always thought sign language might be a universal language, but no, each language has its own form of this. So maybe the language of nature—of the glaciers, rivers, and rocks—is the only universal one.

one could really tell me why. "Girl is distraction," one Sherpa told me, which seemed about as honest of an answer as I was going to get. The Sherpas called me "Lady Climber" and generally expected me to need help with my pack and my crampons until weeks had passed and I showed them I was there to work too. They started teaching me dirty words, not telling me what they meant but laughing when I said them. I started to feel like less of an outsider and more like someone who was supposed to be there.

I began learning the Sherpas' names and movements and grace. I wanted to absorb it all and let the place become part of me. Tshering Dorje and Chhewang Nima were two experienced guides who spoke good English, and they both immediately made me feel welcome. They were funny and strong, and seemed to genuinely enjoy their time on this big mountain. Tshering had the round belly of a Buddha that betrayed his strength. He was quiet and had sweet dark eyes that glowed with care. Chhewang was tall (for a Sherpa) and had the athletic body of someone who practiced fast movement in the mountains. He had a slightly lazy eye and a huge smile with straight teeth and an ever-present laugh. I forced my way into their world and soaked in all they would share.

On the morning of May 8, a jet flew close to the summit of Everest and cheers and hollers spread through all the camps. The Chinese team carrying the Olympic torch had summited, and we were finally allowed to climb higher. Our team was already at Camp Two, so we planned to ascend the Lhotse face the next morning and touch Camp Three before descending to rest for our summit push. All of a sudden, after over a month in Nepal working our way closer, it was happening. I was filled with nerves and the anticipatory excitement of something you really want and the awareness that it might actually happen.

Dave, Mike, and I climbed up to Camp Three and returned to Base Camp that same day, feeling strong and agile in our team of three. We rested for a few more days and headed back up, hoping to see the summit pyramid that had been in hiding for months. I imagined that Everest had a secret she wanted to tell me, but I had to get close to hear it. I shut my mouth and opened my ears as we moved closer and closer. I didn't want to get too excited for fear that it would all slip away, but a buzz of elation was building. I had climbed up to 23,000 feet on Mount Everest. Even if we didn't get to the summit, that was pretty amazing. I had come so far, and I tried not to let the fear of all that was ahead steal that feeling of accomplishment. My Patagonia jacket had traveled from the Four Seasons hotel and now was on its way to Camp Four on Mount Everest.

Camp Four was in the death zone. It was the final camp before the summit, and my highest point ever, at 26,000 feet at the South Col of Mount Everest. Once we attached our oxygen masks, food suddenly sounded good again, seasoned with the fresh and plentiful oxygen flowing through our lungs and saturating our blood and brains. Dave listened on the radios as other climbers went for the summit. It was our plan to rest for a day at the high camp, wait for some of the other people to climb, and then go. We had plenty of oxygen, and the weather forecast promised clear skies. The winds would stay below thirty miles per hour, the cutoff to safely climb.

As we attempted to rest on the night of May 22, the tension at Camp Four escalated as word of the first people of the season making it to the summit from the south side was relayed over broken radio chatter. There was something about hearing that others were on top that made you feel like you were in the wrong place, that you had chosen the wrong date. It became even more tense as day turned to night, and climbers were still descending, out far too long at this very high altitude and almost certainly running out of oxygen by now. I knew it was possible that we would have to forgo our summit push if there was a rescue and we could be helpful. It felt selfish, but I really hoped we wouldn't be faced with that.

We tried to sleep a few hours, waking at eleven p.m. to start getting dressed for our trip to the top. Everything seemed to move in slow motion at this extreme altitude. The lack of oxygen and the extreme cold meant it took twenty minutes to simply put on our boots, and we needed to rest afterward before moving on to the crampons. Another team came over and told us that three people had been out all night, and if we had extra oxygen, we should bring it. My heart was racing with all that was unknown ahead of us. We had a job to do, and to make it work would require constant forward movement.

We secured our masks and goggles and swaddled our bodies in the fluffy down suits that gave us anonymity and protection from the elements. I wondered if Everest would be able to tell that I was a woman, maybe only through my movement, through the energy escaping my feet. We left the camp a few hours after we had woken, finally climbing farther into the thin air.

The first part of the climb from the South Col is steep: a jagged triangular face filled with rock and ice that bursts up from the flat camp for almost a thousand vertical feet before it eases slightly at a bench known as the Balcony. The climbing is so steep that if you lean slightly forward, your face will touch the slope. At two in the morning, my headlamp illuminated the area around my feet as my exhaled breath froze to my mask, making a beard of icicles. The darkness was all-encompassing, with only the bobbing headlamps ahead and behind to break it up. The stars were closer than imaginable but the darkness between them felt truly infinite. I moved in rhythm with Dave. He was in front with Tshering Dorje, Mike next, and me in back. I looked to the right and saw an uneven pile of snow just above me. As we moved closer, I illuminated the lump of snow, noticing now that it had white waxy fingers.

It was a body.

One of the many landmarks on the lower slopes of summit day, it was Scott Fischer, whose dying story is told in *Into Thin Air*. He, too, was a guide. He had died on the descent in horrific storm conditions, and at the request of his family, his body remained entombed on the mountain. I shivered at the sight, somehow both shocking and expected. I considered that people—people like me—died doing this. My own death felt like a distant threat, but this body brought it slightly closer. We kept moving and as we approached the top of the lower third, the sun began to rise, illuminating the peaks below us and the one remaining summit above—Everest. We could see the climbers ahead, and there were many. Dave turned to tell Mike and me that he thought it was unlikely we would get to the top with so many people, but we should keep moving, as we had all season. The weather was perfect, with nearly no wind, but at this altitude it was deadly cold. We checked how much oxygen each person had, and I broke all the icicles from Mike's mask, trying to find my value as a guide while feeling wildly out of my comfort zone. But then, this wasn't supposed to be my comfort zone. I was here to grow.

We moved up the Southeast Ridge above the Balcony, climbing over the steep and jagged rocks barely covered by snow. There were four strands of fixed rope hanging twisted together, making a clump as thick as a fire hose, dangling over the rocks and looking various degrees of weathered and worn. We clipped into as many as would fit into the pear-shaped carabiners attached to our harnesses, unsure what was secure up here in the thin air. Our pace slowed as we caught a large group of climbers who were barely moving. It was difficult to find places where we could safely unclip from the rope and pass other climbers, so we moved slowly in our spot until we could pass. I looked out over the Tibetan Plateau, surprised how it quickly turned from snow to a sandy dry tundra. I looked out to my left, at the high peaks that made up the landscape of Nepal. They all seemed so small and far below us now. I wondered if the mountains ever gazed down at us and marveled at how tiny we were cradled underneath their giant shoulders. We kept moving, one step and one long rest. Repeat. One step. One rest. Time slowed to the speed of our steps, just inching by, step by step. We made it to the south summit. Only the Hillary Step and the long ridge to the summit remained. We tucked into the tiny table-size platform on the south summit and waited for some of the other climbers to descend. Once there was a small clearing, we started again.

It was going to happen. We were going to get to the summit of Everest. I had truly not believed it was going to happen until now. With the final ridge in front of me, I felt the gentle whisper of Everest in my ear as I got closer. The sun shone down on the jewels of ice and reflected her riches back up to me. *You belong here,* I heard her say. I took the final steps to the top. I could see the tops of all the mountains that had once towered over me. I could see the horizon bend around the orb of the earth. Setting down my backpack and looking around, I thought how I had climbed to the tops of the trees as a child, wanting so badly to travel to places I could see from up there. Now I felt the warm embrace of the mountain and I made a silent promise to her: *I won't let you down. I do belong here, and I will make it my home.*

I helped Mike exchange his empty oxygen tank and I tightened his crampons for the descent. Dave hugged me warmly and congratulated me on my first summit. We took photos with the banners Mike carried to the top. I said thank you into the sky, loud enough for everyone to hear, and we descended. As I crossed the exposed rocks surrounded by snow below the summit, I leaned down and slipped a stone in my pocket. I silently promised that I was only borrowing it, and I would bring it back.

After three more days of descending, we made it to Base Camp. We spent a few days packing and cleaning up before beginning the trek down. As we left camp for the final time, everything seemed new and different. I was sure that I wasn't changed just by climbing a big mountain, but I felt somehow different. We stopped for a final cup of dudchia in the first teahouse we came to. On the windowsill was a copy of *Into Thin Air.* I asked the owner if it belonged to someone. He said no, I could take it. So, as we descended from a climb—the climb I always said I didn't want to do—I finally read a book I said I already had.

It felt interesting to read someone else's journey and compare it to what we had just done. I wondered what book would have been written by Charlotte Fox or Sandi Pitman. I wondered if the story of a woman's climb would ever be told. I thought about the joke "Why aren't there more women on Everest? Because women are smarter than that." I was now sure that it had nothing to do with how smart we are. To get to the summit once you must be lucky. To go back again and again, you must be lucky and clever. To learn the lessons of the mountain, you must get there first. And that climb might be the hardest one. But I was here, and as I stood soaking in the possibilities, I never wanted to leave.

* * *

I returned to Rainier and a summer of guiding to make up for the income I hadn't made working on Everest. I returned to the on-again off-again relationship with Brad and the anguish it was causing me. When we all returned to Kathmandu, he showered me with more of the familiar compliments as he tried to flip me back into being his compliant girlfriend. But it didn't matter. The glow of his praise had worn dull, and I could stand on my own away from him. He had made it to the summit, but so had I.

All the other guides on Rainier congratulated me on my summit and asked me for stories of how it was. A freshman class of new guides arrived and began the initiation into becoming mountain gods. There was a Jake and a John and another Rob, just like all the seasons before. There was Tyler, who came with his girlfriend, Katy, who would be a guide too. Tyler was assigned to be my assistant on climb after climb, and he endured hearing my stories of Everest told repetitiously to the clients. The whole time, my mind was distracted with the possibility of returning to Everest, and how I could make that happen. I had so much, but all I wanted was more.

I signed the contract to work as a sponsored athlete for Eddie Bauer, giving me reliable income and snagging the attention of media interested in the brand's chosen representatives. I was tasked with helping to test and build outdoor gear and then take that gear on expeditions and return with beautiful images that would help sell the gear. I was rewarded with expedition funding and a regular paycheck far exceeding what I could make as a mountain guide. Peter was the head of the team, and I dutifully resumed my position as an assistant to him despite my former promise to distance myself. He congratulated my summit, but I could see the envy in his eye. He wanted what I had; I recognized the look as though it was a mirror. He had spent a lifetime trying to get to the summit, and here I was, a twenty-four-year-old woman holding the title he prized.

Peter organized trips for our newly formed team to test new products in South America before heading together to Everest to relaunch the brand's authentic outdoor roots. I was ecstatic for a chance to go back to Everest, and I could feel my professional life ascending, buoyant with opportunity.

But my personal life was falling apart.

After returning from Everest and starting a summer of work back on Rainier, Brad and I continued the rhythm of our dysfunction. He said he wanted to have a family, but he continued to openly question what kind of mother I would be. I resented his power to make me question my own abilities to care for a child in the ways that I had wanted to be cared for when I was small. Finally, the strain of Brad's and my misaligned lives and desires burst and we broke up for good in the middle of the summer Rainier season. I had tried to end it permanently before, but it had become clear to me that I didn't know how to just walk away and be done. I feared that I would again make up with him and smooth it over just to resecure the feeling of belonging to someone. So I executed a move I had been practicing from childhood. I threw a grenade at the relationship and destroyed any chance of it surviving. I agreed to marry someone else.

10.

SOMEONE ELSE'S CLIMB

2009: Mount Everest, Nepal

The further from Everest I got, the more I was sure I needed to go back. Summiting Everest had given me automatic respect among my peers, clients, and strangers seated next to me on an airplane. No matter what you thought I was capable of, I had proven that I could climb the highest peak in the world. Even better, I could guide it! What could prove more that I belonged than that?

I knew what could: On our climb the previous spring, during a rest break in a village below Everest Base Camp, a trio of climbers had arrived to share the teahouse with us for the night, and one of them was a woman. Not just a woman. A warm, beautiful, graceful woman. Her cheeks were pink with the kiss of the sun from time spent up high, and her smooth brown hair was held neatly back with a headband. Gerlinde Kaltenbruner was a famous Austrian alpinist, on a quest to become the first woman to climb all fourteen 8,000-meter peaks, including Everest, without oxygen. She was an actual badass, but somehow still one of the nicest people I had ever met. She spoke quietly and asked us questions about our expedition, and I was enamored by her presence.

So far, my only climbing role models were men. I had decided that women were competition, and you couldn't trust them. I had very few female friends because of this view. And to be fair, Gerlinde wasn't going to become my friend or even my mentor. We were separated by a lifetime and an ocean. But she would become my inspiration. Her journey planted a seed in my mind: What if *I* could climb without oxygen? Then I would stand far apart from the crowds. I could quiet the chatter about only being on the expedition because the client wanted a cute girl there, or because I was the other guide's girlfriend. I could have my accomplishment and do it all on my own. As soon as the thought crossed my mind, I committed to it fully. I *would* do it. I had no idea what it would take, but I was committed mentally. I would learn and I would do it.

As Peter worked with the Eddie Bauer team to pull together an expedition to Everest to launch the outerwear line we had been working on, I voiced my intentions. I wanted to be on the team, and I wanted to climb without oxygen. Peter bristled at this. He wanted to get to the summit, that was the most important thing. After failing twice on previous expeditions, he wasn't looking for anything, or anyone, to interfere with his success this time. But as the team formed and Ed Viesturs agreed to return to Everest as well, Peter happily handed me off to Ed. "The two of you can pursue that goal. The rest of us will climb." It was clear in the way he said "pursue that goal" that he didn't think I could do it.

The Eddie Bauer team had embarked on a series of practice expeditions prior to our April departure for Everest. The first was a trip to Ecuador, attempting to climb one of the 19,000-foot volcanoes that I had first visited with Brad three years before. I was called the team leader on paper, but it was sort of a joke, because Peter led every hike and conversation and, eventually, the climb. The team was made up of five guides and two clients—the CEO of Eddie Bauer and his right-hand man, and a photographer and videographer to capture it all and create content for the brand. Ian was the videographer.

He immediately caught my eye. Ian was everything that Brad wasn't, just as Brad was everything Noah hadn't been. He was calm, rooted, and Scottish. He was nineteen years my senior, and occasionally this age gap seemed to offer me the maturity and stability I craved in my life at that moment. He had youthful but rugged looks with a crop of messy brown hair that always seemed to sit just right. His eyes sparkled with the curiosity of a child as he pursued a life of play, somehow making it into a sustainable profession.

Our flirtation got me reprimanded by Peter within the first few days of the trip, and in my embarrassed resentment I decided to prove to him that this wasn't just me giving attention to someone other than him; it was the real deal.* I didn't know Ian's middle name or that he was known as a forever bachelor. I didn't know where his little condo was in Idaho. But it didn't matter. He was in front of me, another stepping stone out of the life I was living.

After the trip to Ecuador, I agreed to meet him in Nepal as our schedules serendipitously converged across the world. He was teaching kayaking courses, and I was going on an expedition with one of my fellow Eddie Bauer teammates in the Everest region.

Brad was actually in Nepal when I arrived. He had just finished guiding an expedition where they didn't get to their summit, and he was super spun out. He was waiting for me at the hotel when I arrived. He wanted to talk about getting back together, but I told him I couldn't— I had agreed to play tennis with a friend. He asked if he could shower in my room since he was at another hotel. I said yes and went to play tennis to help with the jet lag.

Before I went out, though, the front desk handed me a message from Ian that said to call him at his hotel, with the room number. I crumpled the note and shoved it inside my duffel and went to play tennis. When I was done, Brad was gone. I showered and took a taxi to Ian's hotel, a

---

* I literally had no idea what "the real deal" would even mean in the context of love, and it would take another six years to find out.

small Tibetan locale tucked into a courtyard beyond the busy streets of Kathmandu. Soon I was smiling to myself as I listened to him speak Nepali and receive the warm greeting of the locals like someone who belonged there. He was gentle and warm and open, toward me and everyone he interacted with. I was so used to Brad's suspicious and guarded nature that being around Ian felt like a true respite.

"Well, I think we are about perfect for each other," he told me as we lounged. "We might as well get married." His words poured out with the turn of his Scottish accent.

We had known each other for two weeks.

He asked so casually that I simply agreed, detonating the bomb that would prevent me from returning to Brad. My life was so unrooted already, with no place to live and few friends after years spent isolated in my relationship with Brad.

Just after his casual proposal, the phone rang in his hotel room. Ian picked up, listened, and handed me the phone—it was Brad asking for me. His voice on the phone shocked me. I was shaking, realizing that I was caught. How had he found me? Had he searched through my bags? He begged me to come talk to him and give him a chance, and I just said no. That was it. When I went back to my hotel room the next day, he had thrown my stuff all over the place before he flew, as planned, back to the U.S. That was the last time we spoke.

It wasn't terribly challenging to move into Ian's condo when we returned to the States. It was an adventure, and I felt like I was growing up and staying childish all at once. He was new and I once again felt loved. His love for me showed other people that I was lovable, and I wanted that more than anything. Life was moving quickly, and I was coasting along for the adventure. If I squinted, it all looked right: By the end of 2008, I had summited Everest for my first time, become a sponsored athlete for a major brand, and gotten engaged. I had an expedition planned to return to Everest, and I was finding my footing in this new life, or at least that was what I wanted people to believe. I wanted to believe it too.

Ian and I spent the winter planning a small spring wedding. I flew to Scotland to meet his family and we drove to Colorado for him to meet mine, as fiancés do before a wedding. As he shared a slideshow of his adventures with my parents, I realized that many of them had taken place before I was even born; he was closer to my parents in age than he was to me. But I hushed the practical problems this raised and leaned into my new identity, even if it was an oversize one that didn't quite fit.

Ian continued to film our practice expeditions in the lead-up to Everest and I began to prepare for my second expedition. My heart ached each night as I fell asleep, and when I looked in the mirror in the morning I would quickly look away. I was moving dutifully through the motions of planning a wedding, being a fiancée, trying to wear this life like it fit. But I knew I wasn't being honest. I knew this was not my life, this was not me. I was pretending to want this life with Ian, but I knew deep inside that it would never work. It wasn't me, but I hoped it was taking me toward the life I wanted. I would protect my own heart as I had before, and I would use this experience to get where I needed to be. I looked at the diamond ring Ian had slipped on my hand. This didn't make me his, I promised. I only belonged to myself, and when the time was right, I would run away and find my next home. But for now, I would massage my chest to ease the heartache at night and then I would look quickly away from my own gaze in the morning. I could do this, even if it wasn't perfect. Maybe it wasn't right, but it was going to have to be right *for now.* I was drawing the battle plans to fight for my-self. But there would be no victory.

* * *

My shoulders hunched under the weight of expectations I knew I couldn't fulfill. The glacier ice felt like Styrofoam under my feet as the spikes of my crampons punctured it, slightly sticking with each step and making it even harder to walk at 22,000 feet on Everest. The air around me was cold as the shadow crossed West Shoulder, making it feel like deep winter—dry and dark and endless. Each step was moving me closer to my team, but further from where I wanted to be. With each step I was dragging the previous year of decisions along in much the same way they had been dragging me. The soft fleece fabric around my neck felt stiff and scratchy. The down jacket on top of that felt like a straitjacket. The feeling of being so uncomfortable in my own skin was turning the softest fabrics into sandpaper.

"Peter, Melissa." I keyed my radio mic, resting on a straight leg with my hip jutted out, the pose of the defiant fifteen-year-old girl I thought I had left far behind. The pack on my back was weighted down with food and fuel and two round oxygen cylinders that would be my life gas on summit day. But that was at least two days away from today, and today had barely begun. We had only been moving uphill for an hour, inching above Camp Two toward Camp Three. My breath was heavy, and my heart was bounding irregularly to the rhythm of my chaotic thoughts. Turn around. *Thump.* Keep going. *Thump.* Turn around. *Thump.* The pattern was pulling me in two directions, one up and the other down.

"Go ahead, Melis," Peter replied. He sounded tense, like he was holding the last bit of breath in his chest. He probably was. This was his chance. He was the leader of the team on his summit bid on Mount Everest—the feat that had escaped him twice. On his first attempt at Everest in the early nineties, his father was the expedition leader and didn't choose him to be on the summit bid. He returned years later, leading his own expedition, but the weather was particularly brutal that season and the summit escaped him again. Now was his time to climb, and no one or nothing was going to get in his way.

It hadn't seemed so perverse when the plan was formed nine months earlier, in the safe harbor and rich oxygen of sea level. Up here now, though, the thin façade had eroded, and it was clear that "any cost" included people's lives. Not people "like" me, but me. I had a serious choice to make. Peter was the one choosing the summit day, which weather was acceptable to climb in, and the teams and what gear they

would bring. All of these seemingly mundane details were the difference between a safe climb and tragedy. And the more any individual
thought solely about their own success, the higher the chance of tragedy. The summit called, but my gut was screaming at me to turn
around. I had a horrible feeling the lesson I had learned on Rainier with
Peter—when Ben and Trixie and Gary and I had nearly plummeted to
our deaths—would be repeated, and maybe I wouldn't walk away this
time.

Peter, Ed Viesturs, and Ian were pushing their way up the mountain
toward their summit day. Peter was single-sighted and, in that view,
forsaking his usual sound decision-making. Ed had spent most of the
season alone in his tent, withdrawn from the social structure of the team.
He would join us for meals and the occasional card game with other
team members. He was supposed to be my mentor on this climb—his
sixth of Everest, and my second. I was planning to make the attempt
without supplemental oxygen and Ed was supposed to show me the way
to do it, but it became clear very early that he was uncomfortable with
this role. I was a child, he seemed to think, and that was one thing he
didn't need more of. His wife was eight months pregnant with his
fourth child while we were here trying to climb. An email from her had
been accidentally slipped into my inbox by the Base Camp manager
who manned our communication. In the exchange* his wife told him
she hoped he was still on track to get home by mid-May, as he had
promised. As I scrolled farther down, my own name caught my eye.
"Melissa won't make the climb without oxygen," Ed had written. "She
just doesn't have the eye of the tiger." His words stung like only the salt
of the truest truth can. Any fight I had in me for this massive goal to
climb without oxygen had been seeping away day by day.

As the leader, Peter had a clear vision of everyone's role on this climb.
We had two teams; one was guiding a single client and the other was

---

* Which I read greedily instead of respecting his privacy and moving it to his inbox.
  Shame on me and my persistent curiosity.

made up of Peter, Ed, and me (plus cameras). The main goal was to get Peter to the summit with the Eddie Bauer flag to launch the new outerwear line that had been built by guides. The unspoken goal was simply to get Peter to the summit at all costs. Peter wanted Ian to follow him with a camera and capture him as the hero he had always wanted to be. But as the expedition reached the one-month mark, after more than two weeks of climbing and returning to Base Camp, their relationship had soured. The closer Peter got to his chance to summit, the more expendable everyone else became. The more expendable Ian felt, the more he argued with Peter's vision. It was a defiant standoff and a battle for power, but it wasn't a surprise. The thin air and long expedition tended to wear down one's tolerance.

I was retreating into myself, trying to spend more time alone. Just a few days earlier, when the tension was high and the tolerance low, Ian had woken me up to an announcement of his own. Our wedding was planned for just over a month after the expedition would end. He was already wearing the wedding band I had purchased for him, as a show of commitment. Our shared tent was overfilled with down jackets, boots, and camera batteries. We were lying next to each other, swaddled in our own sleeping bags, when he sat up and slid the little gold ring off his finger and handed it to me. I was barely awake, but knew what was next. "I cannot do this," he said. I didn't question what he meant.

In the weeks before the expedition started, Ian and I had arrived in Nepal so he could acclimatize and be ready to film. It had only been six months since we started dating and five months since we had gotten engaged, but the honeymoon phase of new love had already worn thin. What had, at the start, seemed like a full and adventurous life that we could share now just seemed like an entire lifetime of differences between us. We shared his condo in Idaho, but not much else.

I had imagined that when two broken people saw each other, you could splice them together to make one whole person. But my and Ian's broken borders were misaligned, and in the months since I had left my nomadic truck life to move into his condo in Sun Valley, more light was shining through those cracks and forcing me to pay attention to what was ahead.

By the time he gave back the ring, we had both lost our tolerance for the illusion. I allowed tears to form and hoped they would hide my relief. I felt the acute pain of rejection, but I also felt the spacious relief that freedom bestows. I had gotten engaged to Ian to prove something, and now, feeling the weight of the ring in my hand, I couldn't even tell who I had been trying to prove anything to. Later that day, I moved quietly to an empty tent that had been used for gear storage and instantly felt more like myself than I had in months.

Sitting in the sun, resting before our summit push could start, I told Peter that Ian and I were going to call off the wedding. "Good. I don't trust him," he said, somehow thinking that how he felt was what I wanted to hear. Ever since the Rainier climb with Peter, when he'd split our groups up and my rope team fell, our relationship had changed. He invited me to be on the Eddie Bauer team but didn't hesitate to remind me that he was in charge. When I summited Everest for my first time, he lauded me and told me, honestly, that he was envious. I had something, the one thing, that he wanted most. When I moved to Sun Valley and started dating Ian, Peter welcomed me as a friend more than an employee. I felt like we were starting to become equals—it wasn't only me needing him anymore; he needed me, too. Even though he was fifty, the friendships that surrounded him seemed shallow to me, and so I took my role as his new friend seriously. But I watched him now with a curiosity that replaced the admiration I once felt. I saw how he put on such a beautiful show, captivating most audiences. I saw how he embraced the notion of being selfish: *If you don't look out for you, who will? And what's wrong with that?* I had spent the previous five years as his understudy, hoping to share the stage with him one day. And that day felt close, but I was starting to wonder if his stage was the one I wanted to stand on. It looked lonely. I no longer could only see what he gained by being guarded and self-focused; I was starting to see what he lost.

Peter had been immediately generous with me, wanting to see me succeed from that first day of guide tryouts all the way until now, on Everest. I had been enough for him, and though he held me to a high standard, he didn't ask me to do anything that felt like crossing a line to stay in his orbit, as so many other men in power had. He showed his own imperfect self, even if at times I wasn't sure he knew it was showing. I had been surrounded so often by people who presented a perfect exterior, and in that way, I felt I wasn't good enough to be with or near them. But not Peter. He was brash and confident but also quick to accept criticism and acknowledge his flaws.

But now, as we finally made our way toward the summit, I was filled with hesitation. With the weight of Everest on Peter's shoulders, I could see that he wasn't thinking of me at all. I felt betrayed, as even through the challenges we had endured, I had always wanted to believe that he was looking out for me, too.

"Go ahead, Melissa," Peter repeated on the radio, as I stood paralyzed by the weight of my own words. I steeled myself, knowing I wasn't talking only to Peter. I was talking to everyone with a radio who wanted to listen to our drama unfold. "I am still not feeling great," I said. "I am going to head back to camp, and I'll check in with you in a few hours." I was feigning illness, but really it wasn't sickness in my stomach, it was my gut.

I exhaled. I had pulled open the emergency exit and jumped. I'd said it—I was turning around. My little war of what to do was over.

I didn't know what would come next. I didn't know if I would be allowed another chance at the summit. But I did feel the tremendous relief that comes with opening the door on a cage I had willingly walked into and finally letting myself out. As I returned to my tent at Camp Two, I felt lighter with each step. It was going to be okay. Maybe I could still try for the summit with the other part of our team.*

---

* I could, and I did. I joined fellow climbers and guides Dave Hahn, Seth, and Kent on a stormy and swift summit day. We did not talk to one another for nearly the whole climb, but we did what we came there to do and returned as the same team that had departed.

With Peter, Ed, and Ian moving farther away from me, I finally started to exhale. I wasn't going to climb without oxygen this year, but I also wasn't going to enter a marriage that I never wanted. I wouldn't be able to share the summit with Peter, but I also wouldn't have to share the summit with Ed, knowing he was judging me as an eyeless tiger. With my radio call, I had begun a return to firmer ground, both on the mountain and in my life.

I spent one night alone at Camp Two and then descended as Peter and the team made their way up to Camp Four at the South Col. The tension of their team was ever present in their voices as Peter called down for weather forecasts and to ask how much extra oxygen there was. The mid-May temperatures are brutally low as the jet stream begins to slip away from the summit and climbing becomes possible, and Peter's team was moving up before the jet had fully left, no doubt in part to help Ed keep his commitment to return by mid-May. As they started their summit day, we could still hear the freight train of wind whipping off the top. They pushed on, hoping the winds would calm when it really mattered. Ed used oxygen. Ian fell behind, getting frostbite on his toes. But Peter pushed on, and the wind slowed just enough to allow him and the rest of the team to stand on the summit, Peter's first and only time. I imagine he felt the weight of the chip he had been carrying on his shoulder fall away, and the buoyancy erased the chaos of the climb.

I crossed paths with him at Camp Two as I headed up with the other half of our team. I ducked into his tent to give him a hug and tell him congrats. "You dodged a fucking bullet with Ian. Get away from him as fast as you can." That was his reply. Their tension had reached a fever pitch as Ian openly questioned Peter's decisions and then fell far behind, jeopardizing the only thing Peter cared about—the summit. I was glad I hadn't been there.

Still, my abdominal muscles clenched in rage and embarrassment. Peter was right about Ian, but hearing that made me feel like a fool. I had started the relationship with Ian partly to prove to Peter that it wasn't just a casual flirtation. To have him speak so harshly about Ian now felt like the fullness of his disapproval from the start was finally crashing down on me. He wasn't offering this like advice to a friend, he was commanding it like a boss. I didn't want to need his approval—that was part of what I was trying to do here, prove that I was good enough, and I didn't need Peter or Ian or Ed to be the one to decide that.

Peter and the rest of his team returned to Base Camp as my team ascended toward our goal. There was a spaciousness in the movements of this new team. The primary goal of getting Peter to the summit was accomplished. I hoped it would heal a wound that he had been carrying for so long, but the words of Dave Hahn, my new team leader, were lingering in my head: "Getting to the summit of Everest never made anyone more humble." Dave had summited Everest fourteen times, the most of anyone who wasn't Sherpa, so he should know. But I wasn't sure he was right. When I had stood on that tiny patch of ice the previous year, my entire body was flooded with a type of humility that made my feet feel light and my body heavy. It reminded me of that first climb, in Montana, where I felt so small and so big all at once.

Ed was already gone by the time we got back to Base Camp, and Peter had stuck around just long enough—at the request of the Base Camp manager—to provide nominal backup and offer a quick congrats before he was gone too. With their absence everything took on a less urgent quality. We still had several loads of gear at Camp Two needing to be brought down, so we rested a day and prepared to finish our work. Ian and I slept in separate tents, not sharing any more space, words, or pretense of love.

Everyone was tired from their respective climbs, and we packed up the two-month-long expedition without any urgency. It was over, we were done, no need to rush away. The days moved slowly as we inched toward our departure day and the return to normal life, or whatever remained of it, which for me was nothing. Dread began to creep in. I would have preferred to keep sleeping in my little tent perched on the ice indefinitely, safely tucked away from all the questions that I knew I would have to answer about my cratered engagement.

On the last night in Base Camp, I was awoken by a deafening silence. It is hard to imagine how silence can wake you, but the complete vacuum of sound was so unsettling that I shot straight up in my tent. Something was wrong. I couldn't see the normal glow of the Base Camp lights that stay on all night. In a moment, I realized what was happening: The tent was about to collapse under an unmanageable amount of snow, nine feet in twelve hours. The fabric was sinking closer to me under the immense weight. I hit the fabric hard, shaking off enough snow to unzip the door and dig my way out.

I crawled out, rushing to put on my boots while shaking off the groggy sleep. I needed to start shoveling the snow off the tents that hadn't collapsed yet and make sure everyone else was awake and out of the tents, too. The camp looked like a series of small snow-covered mountains, strangely calm with the muffled quiet from the snow. The silence was quickly replaced by anxious clamor as the camp came alive with the activity of digging and packing hastily. Everything that was still at the upper camps was buried and positioned under avalanche slopes, making it inaccessible. There was no more sleep that night, only digging out tents and quickly packing away the final items for retreat at first light. The mountain was rushing our exit. We fled Base Camp in a militant line.

Ian and I didn't speak again until we sat together in Kathmandu composing an email to our wedding guest list, informing them that they were now free on June 29. And we were free, too. I had made it to the summit of Everest for my second time, but the climb felt like someone else's. I wanted a do-over. I not only wanted to find the eye of the tiger that Ed said I didn't have, but I also wanted to be the tiger. I wanted to be capable and dominant and respected.

Before boarding the plane home from Kathmandu, I already had started planning for the next season. I had already started moving on in the well-practiced way of the woman I was becoming. I had a year. In a year I could become a tiger. I could plan an expedition. It would be small, only Dave Morton and myself. I could exist in discomfort to prepare for the challenge of an oxygen-free climb. I could be brave enough to be alone for the first time in my adult life.

11.

EXILE

2009: Sun Valley, Idaho

Back in Sun Valley for the summer, I was ready to begin training to climb Everest without oxygen, but I was unprepared for the consequences of ending my engagement to Ian.* I trudged through the logistics of canceling the wedding venue, the caterer, the flowers, shame accompanying each call. I felt like everyone expected this after a hasty engagement to a man I barely knew. I was scared to go to the grocery store, fearing someone would ask me when the wedding was.

As the canceled wedding day got close, the emotion of it caught me

---

* The 2009 expedition had been funded by Eddie Bauer as a launch of the First Ascent line of technical outerwear that we had spent the previous year building. When I returned, I met with the CEO and suggested to him that I wanted to go back to Everest. He said he would support my goals and he was sure I could do it. I appreciated the belief and support and proceeded with my planning.

by surprise, even though it was a day I was sure I didn't want. I looked at my wedding dress, pure white chiffon layers with a draping open back, hanging on a lonely hanger in my new condo. Losing a thing I hadn't really wanted still seemed to create a void.

My sister and her husband had taken time off from work to attend my wedding, but since the wedding was off, they decided to instead meet my parents at a Montana lake for a weekend of camping. Without the obligation, they were free to gather without me. It didn't come as much of a surprise that I wasn't invited.

My sister and I had an icy relationship in high school after the move to Montana, but in the years since we had both moved out of our parents' house we had reconnected as friends. I admired her drive and the way she kept the same job and the same friends for what seemed like forever. She was anchored in all the ways that I was transient, but there was still a secret language of knowing that we both spoke. We had come from the same place, and there were things we would never have to describe to each other. She became my closest family member, and the one I would check in with when things were either good or bad.

But in the almost ten years that had passed since I moved out of my parents' house, I had barely spoken to them. Christmas, birthdays, a hello here or a congratulations and what's new there. Meanwhile, my parents and my sister were friends with one another. They were family. I was a stranger to my parents, although they were starting to know a little more about my life from the media covering my Everest career, and they complimented my interviews and congratulated my accomplishments as a fan would. They had distantly supported my hasty engagement, accepting that there must be much about my life that they didn't know. I shared with them only what I would share with an acquaintance. Superficial and safe. I guarded myself in every interaction, calculating what to say and how to say it. I was scared that if I allowed them into my life in any meaningful way, they would destroy it as I had once destroyed theirs.

It was easier to keep them at a distance. My dad occasionally reached across the chasm and offered a hug of genuine love or deeper curiosity as to how I was doing. He asked questions and gave praise. "I am so proud of you, Miss," he said when I talked about my guiding work. "You are living the life I always wanted. When I joined ski patrol, that was my happiest time, and now that is your life." His soft eyes were wet with emotion. He was proud of me, and I could feel it. I tried reaching back, but it broke my heart more than it mended it. His was a love I couldn't fully accept. I feared that it might be ripped away, much like it had been before. I was afraid of holding him hostage in the impossible distance between me and my mother, threatening to make him choose. I was afraid he wouldn't choose me.

Even though I wasn't invited to the family gathering, I decided to make the four-hour drive to the lake in Montana. I already felt so uncomfortable in my life, I figured I may as well submerse myself in the most discomfort possible and hope it could be a distraction. As I drove, I listened to Ani DiFranco and sang out loud. I cried warm, wet tears as I cruised through a desolate stretch of highway snaking alongside the river. How had I allowed myself to get to this point? How had I allowed myself to be so publicly rejected with the announcement of a canceled wedding? How would I rise from this and prove that I was not the disaster I saw when I looked closely at myself? I could easily hide behind my summits and pretend I was successful, but I knew it was a lie.

I arrived late in the evening, to the surprise of everyone but my sister, who had told me where they were going. I quickly drank a beer, then another one, as they peppered me with questions about Everest. I felt worn down, and the canceled wedding day was shining a bright light on my feelings of failure. My dad told me I looked older. He stood tall, with his same long beard, now peppered with gray. His face was weathered but his eyes had remained kind despite all the heartache over the years. He was working as a building inspector in a small town in

Colorado and had recently taken up trail running, and his body showed the strong sinewy muscles of an athlete. I stood near him and the slight comfort he provided. He loved me, he always had, and I knew that. For some reason this now made me feel sad, unworthy of his kindness, and I fought back tears.

"Why the pout?" my mother asked, nodding her chin toward my body, which I had collapsed against the campsite's wooden picnic table. I tensed as she spoke to me, not quite knowing how to interact with her. I felt like a child, both scared and helpless and then frozen. She too had a weathered face, the wrinkles of a smoker carved deep around her lips. Her hair was thin, the same dishwater brown, worn in the same shoulder-length style with a thin curtain of bangs. She had a new limp from some sort of hip pain. I imagined it must be the hurt inside her, still finding physical ways to leak out.

She had listened as I talked about Everest, but this was the first sentence she had spoken directly to me. And to be fair, I hadn't talked to her either. I had spoken in her direction, but I avoided eye contact and direct exchanges at all costs. That was how we had learned to interact, a compromise to keep the peace. I exhaled and let the warm swaddle of the beer remove my carefully cultivated inhibition. "It is supposed to be my wedding tomorrow." My shoulders shrugged into my ears and stayed there as I slouched farther over. My voice cracked, threatening to reveal more than I had wanted to. If I showed weakness, or emotion, I feared she would attack.

"You have a job. You climbed Everest two times. Your life isn't so hard." Her tone was cold, slightly mocking. She took a long drag of her cigarette as she volleyed her words at me with intention. "I am surprised you didn't go through with it, though. I assumed you would marry an older man."

This was an accusation. I disguised my discomfort in a short laugh and a long sigh. What could I possibly say? I looked at her and could only see the shattered past that had brought us here. She still thought it was all my fault. We were strangers verging on enemies and she thought that everything that had brought us here had been my choice. How could she forget that I was a child then and that she wasn't the only one who lost something?

* * *

I opened another beer, stood, and said goodnight, crawling a few moments later into the safe confines of the back of my truck. I took a sleeping pill and drank the beer as I nestled into my sleeping bag. I closed my eyes, covering them with my palms as hot tears forced their way out. Seeing my family thrust me back in time. As much as I wanted to escape my memories of how it all started, they were ghosts that would persistently show up uninvited. I wondered if I welcomed the harsh discomfort of climbing Everest without oxygen because I had become so accustomed to discomfort that I liked its familiarity. Maybe I deserved to be uncomfortable. Maybe if I chose it before it chose me, it would feel like a reward, not a punishment.

As sleep teased my brain, I saw his face. It had been years since he had shown up behind my closed eyes. He wasn't welcome, and I did my best to keep him out. But he was here now. His face looked gentle, but I couldn't trust my memory anymore. Had it been gentle or calculating? I saw him reaching out and hugging the shadow of my twelve-year-old self. I heard his words: "I will come find you." It felt like a promise more than a threat. Now, thirteen years later, I still wondered if he would.

The beer and sleeping pill worked against my mind as it wandered back to that time, to the Friday my parents were coming home to a ruined trailer.

There was a small parrot. It had a cage, but the door was always open, and the bird flew freely around the room, landing occasionally to peck on a wooden picture frame. The mother in the foster house was named Bess. She was round and gentle with long, braided brown hair and ruddy pink cheeks like I imagined Mrs. Claus must have. She showed me the room where I would stay, leading me to the bed to set down my school backpack, the only item I had with me. Even the books inside weren't mine. I wondered where my sister was. I wondered where my parents were. I wondered why I had thought that everything would be okay.

I sat down on the little twin bed with the floral cotton bedspread and single flat pillow. Bess left to give me some space, pulling the door shut with a quiet click. I heard her walk back to the living room, where Jane, the social worker, was waiting patiently while I got settled in my temporary foster home.

I felt the shaky flood of adrenaline in my body starting to settle. It was only four o'clock, but I was exhausted. I didn't know what to do in this little room that wasn't mine. There was a big computer on a little desk. There was a little window. Maybe I could jump out of it. But where would I even go? I decided to take a nap, and then I could plan my escape. I slid off my white sneakers and lay down on the bed. I hadn't napped in as long as I could remember. I flipped over, lying on my stomach and tucking my arms underneath me in a protective position with all my vital organs hidden. I felt the hollow curves of my skinny child's body. It didn't make sense to me, this child's body. I was all grown up now and it felt wrong to occupy the innocent form of a kid.

It was officially the longest week of my life. I had lived an entire life's worth of emotions. I was scared. I was hopeful. I was sad. I was a mix of all the things I couldn't even understand. The avalanche had started the previous weekend, but the snow had been building up, unstable and ready to release, for much longer than that. Just one week ago, as I was waiting for the bus, Officer Jones had come to talk to me. I had felt all the cells in my body begin to vibrate the way they always did when he approached or when I saw his turquoise Chevy pickup in the school parking lot. I loved him. I was in love with him. He was going to take care of me, and I was going to get to live the life I had always wanted. With him. That was what he told me.

I wanted to be loved so badly, and here he was, willing to do it. I thought about my mother, and how I wanted her to love me, too, but my wanting it had never made it happen and I was sure it never would. To have his love, I would need to remove the obstacle of my parents.

The door of the foster house bedroom creaked open. I turned from the bed to see a young girl of about six or seven. I heard Bess, the foster mom, coming down the hall. "Leave her alone, sweetie. She needs some space."

The little girl didn't move. She had a hairbrush in her hand, and clear, bright blue eyes. "My name is Hope. Will you braid my hair?" she asked, extending the brush in my direction. I took it from her and nodded. I realized with shocking speed and weight that my life wasn't going to be what I thought it was at all. All I had was this room that wasn't mine, a hairbrush, and Hope.

After I eventually returned to my parents' house, after the social worker required our family to attend counseling together, after my mother had refused to return beyond the first session and said I was "fucking crazy, a pathological liar"—after all that, for months on end, I wasn't spoken to about anything but the logistics of life. I spent most of my time in my bedroom, writing in my journal and fantasizing about running away to be with Officer Jones. I was lonely and alone and trying to understand a world much bigger than my twelve-year-old brain and heart could comprehend. I did run away. Twice. But I was caught and returned to my parents both times. And then one day, my parents moved us to Montana.

I wasn't the only one Officer Jones had been taking out of class, I learned. There was a high school junior, sixteen, and now she was pregnant with his child. My heart was broken as I saw her living the life he had promised to me. I had given up everything I knew in my life. I had betrayed my family and severed any chance of normalcy because I believed that I would be with him and I would be safe and loved. I was only twelve and I couldn't yet imagine how life worked, but I could imagine a love story with a happy ending. This was not it. He was supposed to save me, not her.* Knowing she would be with him was heartbreaking.

In my own home, my mother reminded me that as soon as I was eighteen and she could legally kick me out,† she would. "You have ruined my life. And as soon as you can get out of my house, you will." Her words were always sharp, suffused with disgust at who I was and how I could possibly be her daughter at all. She said that I was a liar. That I was garbage. That I was less than garbage. I kept silent. There was nothing left to say.

Montana was supposed to be a clean slate, but it still showed the dirty chalk dust of what had been done. My sister would barely talk to me. My mother didn't talk to me. My father would reach for me only when no one was looking, offering me a reminder of what I had lost. His love pained me, and so I resisted it. I didn't deserve it anyway. At the new school in a new state, a new teacher started taking me out of class. I wondered if this was just what adult men were going to do with me forever. Groom me to trust them and trick me into feeling loved by someone with power. Lure me in with the promise of the care I was missing and then use me in any way they wanted to. I entered a deep sadness. I wanted a different life. One where I wouldn't have to rely on anyone but myself, the only person I could really trust.

* * *

In the back of my truck, by the lake in Montana, the sleeping pill wasn't working. Even after all this time, my family still only tolerated me. I told myself that I didn't care. I didn't need them. I didn't need Officer Jones or Ian or Brad, or Peter. I didn't need anyone. I was going to rise

---

* I really saw it then as him saving me. Which is heartbreaking to think now.

† She would threaten it all the time, saying she wasn't going to let me live in her house one day longer than the law required.

above it all, all by myself. I shifted my mind back to the slopes of Everest. The challenge there was nothing compared to what I had already survived. I breathed deeply, imagining going back and climbing all the way to the summit without oxygen. I imagined returning to Base Camp, the first American woman to complete the challenge. I imagined all the love I would get. I could replace these horrible memories with new ones and rewrite the story of my life.

12.

FULL MOON

October 2010: Baruntse, Nepal

The trail we took that fall wasn't the one we had intended to walk. It wasn't even Plan B. It was more like the last alternative in a series of plans that hadn't gotten off the ground. In my frantic desire to salvage any expedition, I had duly ignored all the signs that were saying *Not now.* I had gotten distracted by looking too far ahead, and now here I was, soaking wet in a tiny mud-walled kitchen, filled with porters who were also soaking wet. We were all choking on the dense smoke of an open fire burning wet wood as we huddled together trying to dry ourselves out.

"Didi, can you come help? This guy is sick." Chhewang ducked his head into the little smoke-filled kitchen. I was the only woman, and the only non-Nepali.

We weren't on the path into Everest Base Camp; in fact, from the airport in Lukla we had walked in the opposite direction, on an obscure route that launched us straight up to 15,000 feet and back down to

11,000 feet in a single day. It was a trail of curiosity for us both—neither Chhewang nor I had spent much time in this valley, but it would lead us to the foot of the peak that we intended to climb: Baruntse—a lesser-known 23,000-foot peak that was starting to interest climbers as a possible training peak for higher Himalayan mountains. Baruntse was an imposing beast of a mountain, hosting a high pass that divided the Khumbu valley from the Makalu valley. My friend Jiban, whom I'd met during my first trip to Nepal with Mike and who had since become a close friend, had arranged the logistics and permits from Kathmandu.* He had also called Chhewang to see if he could join me.

I had known Chhewang for a few years at this point. We had worked alongside each other on Everest and then on Rainier, but I had really gotten to know him the previous year during a summit of Ama Dablam, a stunning 22,000-foot peak in the Everest valley. Chhewang was exceedingly well-liked and respected among both foreigners and Sherpas. He had summited Everest nineteen times, the second most of any human after Apa Sherpa, who had twenty summits. He lived in a little village tucked into the hills below Everest, where he and his wife farmed potatoes, herded yaks, and raised his two preteen boys when he wasn't working on expeditions or traveling to the U.S. in the summer.

Chhewang was now a well-known and respected guide, but he came from incredibly humble beginnings. He had grown up in another, smaller village just up the valley in a big family with eight kids and hundreds of yaks. He began his climbing career as a porter and was eventually allowed on an Everest expedition by an uncle who was the Sherpa leader, called a Sirdar. His first time in the Khumbu icefall humbled him, showed him the physical strength he lacked. He didn't know

---

* Jiban had become a friend in the years since I met him on my first Everest expedition. He was one of a hundred different Nepali agents who you could book logistics through, and in my observation, he was the best. He was able to make things happen when no one else could, and I had taken to calling him Don Jiban, a nod to a guy with all the right connections.

how to properly put on his harness or his crampons. His uncle kept his secret and showed him the way. Chhewang summited that season, and his life was forever changed. He would be a mountain worker. His charisma and willingness to learn English made him a natural with foreign clients, who were always quick to connect with him. His distinct smile and one lazy eye made him easy to recognize.

Chhewang's bright smile and funny jokes were a nice reprieve from the generally serious nature of the other Sherpas. I joked with him that first year that if I ever needed to find him it was easy—I just had to follow the laughter of the other Sherpas and he would be there. He was kind to me, and he also respected that I was there to do a job, the same job as him. We had bonded not long after we met when he stood at the door of the tent as I spent seventy-two hours caring for a Sherpa who had been poisoned by bootleg liquor. He understood then that I wasn't just expecting the Sherpas and porters to take care of me; I was there to take care of them, too.

Our friendship had truly blossomed the next year on the Ama Dablam expedition, a mission to collect photos for Eddie Bauer. Our small team consisted of me and Chhewang and my friend Cory, a skilled mountain photographer and climber. We had rejected a multistage expedition-style climb in favor of a single-push alpine-style one,[*] making our whole trip less than two weeks, which had cemented the idea that we could climb in a similar style on Dhaulagiri, an 8,000-meter peak. But that summer, as we were planning and preparing for the trip, Cory had hurt his back in a climbing accident. I had already bought my tickets to Nepal, so I began to scramble for another trip. I found one guiding a trek into Everest Base Camp and I asked Jiban to ask

---

[*] Alpine style is considered to be the purest form of climbing, where you climb a mountain from the bottom to the top in a single push, without climbing up higher and fixing rope to the route and setting camps (as in expedition style). It is riskier, as there is more unknown, and you exchange the usual exploration of the route ahead with speed to stay safer.

Chhewang if he maybe wanted to climb Baruntse after he got done leading a trek of his own. He said he did, and we planned to meet after a few
weeks, in the middle of October.

Now we were here, a few days into the weeklong walk to the Base
Camp of Baruntse, soaking wet after a full day of rain and snow. "The
rain comes when they kill the animals in Kathmandu, Meli Didi," Chhewang shared as he slurped spicy ramen noodles, addressing me in the
nickname he chose, Meli, and the sweet Nepali addition of "big sister."
Even though I was his little sister—or bahini—by age, it was more re-
spectful to call me Didi, and he always did. "The Gods get angry; it always rains when the festival season happens." There were Hindu festivals
in late October each year, some including animal sacrifice. I listened,
wondering if he was right.

It was just the first night of our trek when Chhewang came into the
kitchen where I was drying my feet by the fire. The concern on his face
was obvious even before he spoke. "This guy very sick. Do you have
some medicine?" I nodded and crouched my way through the low doorway and into the rain. My backpack was underneath baskets full of potatoes and ramen noodles carried by the porters, and I had to dig through
them, squinting in the fading light of a fast-approaching night. I pulled
out my headlamp and first-aid kit and followed Chhewang back inside
and into another small room, the one we would sleep in that night.
Twelve mats covered the floor, slightly spaced from one another, and a
pile of cheap Chinese fleece blankets sat in the corner. Just inside the
dark space were two men, both small with crooked bodies burdened by
years of carrying loads too heavy for any human. Nepali people aren't
very tall in general (except Chhewang, at about five-nine—a giant by
Sherpa standards), but porters who carry heavy loads are even smaller
and more hunched by the weight of a hard life and a job that crushes
them closer to the earth each day.* One man was standing, and the other

* The porters are a lifeblood of this region, not just for tourists. In Lukla, at 9,000 feet,
there is no more motorized transport to connect almost a hundred villages. When

was cradled inside a basket that was typically used to carry goods. There were holes cut out for his legs and he was hunched over, resting his torso on a rolled-up pad. I could hear the alternating gurgle and wheeze of his attempts to breathe, and I immediately felt helpless, knowing what was ahead. I talked to the men, with Chhewang translating, and discovered he had been sick from the altitude for a few days. But in the last few hours he developed this cough, and then he kept passing out. Now he couldn't even talk.* They gave him aspirin but didn't have anything else or know what else to do.

I could tell by the noises that accompanied the labor of each breath that he had high-altitude pulmonary edema, or, put simply, fluid-filled lungs—a very bad sign. I asked Chhewang if he thought there was oxygen anywhere in the village and he said no. I listened to gurgles of fluid in the man's lungs as I read his oxygen saturation with a small tool I kept in my first-aid kit for times exactly like these—44 percent. A reading below 80 percent in an urban environment would be considered catastrophic. Here in the high mountains, 80 percent was acceptable, but people started to feel bad and show it when the numbers dipped below 75 percent. Forty-four was nearly dead. At this point, there was little left to do for him.

I stepped outside with the other porter and Chhewang. "I have some medicine that we should give him," I said, "but it might be too late." Even with the medicine, he needed to get down below the 11,000 feet of this village to have any chance at survival. It was dark now and still raining. The only way down to a lower altitude was up the 15,000-foot pass first and then down to 9,000 feet, and it would take more than twelve

---

people need supplies, they rely on porters to bring them, whether that is food or building materials. The entire area is built, literally, on the backs of these men.

* The porters are often from low-elevation tribes, and they don't naturally acclimatize as well as the Sherpas do, so altitude issues aren't uncommon. Some porters are Sherpa, but mostly they come from other tribes.

hours for someone to try to carry the man all that distance. And even then, without oxygen on the way, he was unlikely to make it.

The man told us he would try anyway and thanked us as I gave him the medicine for his friend. Chhewang and I went back to the smoky kitchen. Chhewang kept touching his tongue against the roof of his mouth, making the click-click noise of a situation that was bad and unfixable. Death in the mountains seemingly came in two ways: abrupt and violent with little warning, or slow and suffocating. I had seen both play out on rescues throughout my years working as a guide, and I had wrapped the notion in the distant thought that death was an inevitable part of life, one none of us could avoid, and it was far better to die while doing something that made you feel alive than be robbed of life while you were distracted by the mundane. But in times like these, I knew deep down that the idea that a death in the mountains was some-how nobler was only a lie I was telling myself to quiet the fear, as well as the selfishness that I felt about pursuing something with such finite consequences.

Within an hour the porter was back. His friend had died, he said. There was no more breath. The other porters welcomed him in, offering no words—just hot tea and homemade booze. I sat in silence with them until our noodles were gone, and then Chhewang and I left to claim a mat for the night. I wondered if this, too, was happening because the animals were being sacrificed in Kathmandu.

* * *

The next day the sun rose, and the electric blue of the sky pushed the clouds away. We continued our journey toward Baruntse, quiet as we walked but sharing stories in the teahouses where we stopped to sleep. "Do you think you will eventually have the most summits of Everest?" I asked him as we shared more noodles. Chhewang's guiding was a notch above many of the other Sherpa guides, and he was starting to receive recognition outside his community. He had recently acquired sponsorship from an apparel company and all eyes were on him each Everest season as he inched closer to holding the record for most summits.

"I want to," he said, offering a coy little smile. "Then I bring my family to the U.S." I nodded, understanding that climbing was freedom for him just as it was for me, though we were escaping different things.

Chhewang's stories were short, and I often had to coerce details from him to better understand. "When you are herding yaks," I asked curiously, "do your yaks go out in the field with other people's yaks, or do you keep them all separate?" I was thinking of cattle and how we brand them to tell who their owners are. I wondered how it worked in the high hills of the Himalayas.

He laughed out loud at my simple question. "No, they all go together. Every family. We maybe have forty and my cousin has fifty. They go together to the fields."

"How do you know which ones are yours?" I asked.

"Ha, you know them by their faces. They grew up in your house since they were babies. You know them." This concept mystified me, that he could remember the faces of so many animals, but he assured me it wasn't amazing at all. I knew where all the letters on the keyboard of the computer were without looking, he noted, which was the same thing. To me, one of those skills was more useful than the other, and it wasn't mine. He tried to explain the elaborate rules of the card game called marriage that the Sherpas liked to play, but it was as foreign to me as the language and the silence that was so abundant. Mostly, we moved together in silence. It struck me that there is such a difference between a comfortable silence and an uncomfortable silence, and I was grateful that ours was one of comfort. For the past year, I had been moving through my days looking for an escape from the discomfort I had created with Ian. I had mostly busied myself with work in the mountains and distanced myself from those who cared about me. And now I was happy to be here with Chhewang, moving simply without any need to know what my life would be like when it was time to go back home.

After a week alone on the trail, we were at the Base Camp of Baruntse, reunited with other Sherpas and a smattering of expeditions. The winds had been high this season, and no one had made it onto the summit ridge yet. Chhewang and I planned to head up to Camp One the next morning, continue to Camp Two the day after, and then see what the weather was doing. That would put us on a similar schedule to his friends who were guiding clients. He wanted to help them fix the summit ropes if he could, which would allow the route to easily be climbed by all of the coming clients. We had helped fix the ropes on Ama Dablam the previous year and I knew he took great pride in opening the route, though it was often a dangerous challenge, as the leader would be breaking through the deep snow, unprotected by their own ropes, to put in the path to the summit.

The next morning, as we packed to head to Camp One, I divided the gear between us equally: a picket for each of us, part of the tent, and a few fuel canisters. As I tucked my load into my bag, Chhewang came over and asked if he could carry some of it. "I am Sherpa, Didi, I am very strong," he said, holding out his hands.

"No! What if something happens to you? I have to know that I can carry all my own things. I am Meli. I am very strong!" I grinned and flexed my arms like a bodybuilder.

He laughed and agreed. "Sherpa know you don't fight with the woman," he said with a smirk. We zipped the doors to the tent we would leave at Base Camp, filled with our duffel bags and extra food that would stay there.

"They are smart," I replied.

"The only thing stronger than Sherpa is a woman's will." We both giggled. He was right.

We traveled through the rocky moraine and crested the first steep and icy slopes to arrive at Baruntse Camp One in good time and tucked in for the night. The journey to Camp Two the next day was a short one but got us just a little closer to the summit. We were feeling good, but the weather wasn't cooperating at all, as the winds continued to batter the mountain. The short journey took much longer than we planned, and when we arrived, we hastily put up our tiny two-man tent and crawled inside, protected. The next twenty-four hours were filled with making water, drinking water, eating noodles, getting out to pee, eating snacks, and starting to get restless as the wind scoured the slopes above and whipped our little tent around.

As the sun dawned and rose on our third day on the mountain, the winds began to fade. Chhewang's friends, a group of three Sherpas, had set up their camp next to us, and they were gearing up to climb toward the upper mountain. There was a Pasang and two Lakpas who all came from the valley just above Chhewang's village. He had worked with them before, but I was meeting them for the first time. "Didi, I go with them and fix the ropes to the summit and then we come back and climb tonight, okay?" He told me his plan matter-of-factly.

I nodded. "I wonder how far you will get?" I was looking out at the flat valley that had to be crossed before gaining the upper mountain. I expected that it would be filled with light snow that would be treacherous to trailbreak their way through. Chhewang secured his harness and put on his shell jacket and backpack and left. I curled up in my sleeping bag and let my mind wander back home, to Idaho and what was waiting for me there.

I had spent the summer single after calling off my wedding to Ian. I moved into my own little condo, a fully furnished rental down the road from his, and I spent most of my time working on Rainier or teaching medical courses to distract me from the reality of a broken engagement and the breakup that followed. He came to my little condo almost weekly with some form of negotiation on how we should give our relationship another go, but I was ready to move on, certain that I didn't want to be stuck in another make-up/break-up cycle like I had been with Brad.

We had managed to keep a distant friendship of sorts through the summer, and as fall came, Ian was also working in Nepal as a river guide. Before I left on my trip, he had asked me to bring him some medicine he had accidentally left in Idaho.* I brought it and we met up for tea on my arrival in Kathmandu. The tea turned into a nostalgic walk down memory lane and the best parts of our relationship. The nostalgia turned into a night spent in his bed and the promise of being together "one last time" before we said goodbye for good.†

I left the next morning for the trek with my clients. On the third day, I checked my email to find a note from Ian, telling me he felt like our going separate ways for good was the right choice and he wished me well.

There was also a message from Jon. I had met him the week before I left Idaho. He was interesting and charming and confident and new. He was closer to my age. He had a strong jaw and jock-ish good looks. He drove a truck identical to mine, and after spending a day paddleboarding on a mountain lake with him I had agreed to stay in touch while I climbed through the Himalayas. He loved following my progress by scouring Google Maps for my destination. He had filled my email inbox with links to songs and funny little notes in a serious effort to not let me forget him. I was curious and I felt like maybe something could be there, but I didn't want to make the same mistakes I always had. If I was going to date him, it wasn't going to be to prove anything or get anything. I wasn't sure if I could open myself up and attempt to be honest and vulnerable.

As I sprawled out in the tent alone, I imagined what getting to know Jon might be like when I got home. Those thoughts faded into sleep, and after a few hours I woke up to a light breeze and a tent that had gotten way too hot. I looked out the door at the slope above. Chhewang and the other three were out of sight. The travel must have been quicker than we thought. I wondered again how high they would go. I

---

* It was a medication he had to take after his open-heart surgery the previous year. If a nineteen-year age difference ever feels small, there is nothing like attending your partner's open-heart surgery to widen that chasm.

† Such a dumb notion.

decided to make a few thermoses of hot tea and soup for them for when they returned.

The snow melted slowly into water and then boiled before I transferred it to the thermoses. As I turned down the stove, I heard the whoops and yells of Sherpas coming down from above. I opened the tent door to see them coming quickly back to the tents. I put on my boots and climbed out with the thermoses to greet them. They were making so much noise that I assumed they must have somehow made it to the summit. I raised the thermoses over my head, one in each hand, beckoning them closer with the promise of hot fluid. Pasang came rushing toward me. "Congrats, Dai! How did it go?" I said jubilantly.

"No!" His words were escalating, and his tone was frantic. "Chhewang Nima all gone. Chhewang Nima finished!" He fell to his knees, hyperventilating into a heap of tears. The other two Sherpas came down to us, moving with less urgency.

"What happened?" I asked as they exchanged words in Sherpa or Nepali. The feeling of doom was closing in on me. My stomach clenched in fear. "WHAT HAPPENED?!" I begged them to speak in English so I could understand.

But words would not allow me to understand the truly unimaginable reality. The oldest of the three spoke slowly, using his hands to show me. They were climbing fast, he said, and getting the fixed ropes in place when the ridge that Chhewang was on suddenly broke free. It was a cornice and it avalanched down the slope toward Makalu, taking him with it. He was gone. There was no sign of him. They had looked and looked, but it was a steep cliff that washed out thousands of feet below. There was no way he survived.

I stood silent, devastated. I could not make my mind believe it. Chhewang was careful and experienced. He knew snow and he wouldn't have been on the slope if it was unstable. This couldn't be happening.

I asked them if we could go back up and look. They said they would in the morning. But now they had to rest. They quickly took off their crampons and crawled, all three of them, into their little tent. I stood there alone. I looked up at the empty slope above, the wind now totally gone. Chhewang wasn't coming back, ever. I got into my own tent, our tent, and felt the weight of this reality start to settle onto me. There had to be a way out of this. Maybe I was dreaming. Maybe if I prayed, he would come back and be fine. He was so strong; he could endure so much. Maybe he would survive the night and we would find him in the morning.

Why did we come here? Why did we have to do this? Nothing had been going right. But I didn't have any bad feelings today . . . Wasn't I supposed to have a bad feeling before something this catastrophic happened? Why him? He was so kind and special and . . . My frantic thoughts raced across my mind, preventing tears from coming. I looked at his sleeping bag. I looked at his phone and a small stuff-sack of extra gloves and clothes. My chest felt hollow and empty in the space where my heart belonged. Was this my fault? Why did we come here? As my thoughts cascaded and crashed into one another, one of the Sherpas opened my tent door. "We are going down. Pasang is in trouble. You come down, too."

He zipped the door and left me to wonder what was happening. It was almost dark. But what else was there to do? What good would it be to sit there alone all night? I could get to Base Camp and my satellite phone, and I could call Jiban and tell him. I packed all my things and used every inch of space I had left to pack all of Chhewang's things. It would be a stretch to fit the tent as well. But if I left it . . . Well, maybe if I left it and he was somehow alive still, he could climb down and have a place to sleep. I emptied the tent of all our things and secured the anchors with my last bit of unrealistic hope.

Pasang was in emotional shock after what he had seen, and he was hysterical, so he was now using the emergency oxygen bottle his team carried for their clients. We descended together by headlamp, clumsy in our grief. Within a few hours, Base Camp came into view. I didn't want to go to the tent full of Nepalis who would be speaking their language while I struggled to understand. I didn't want to make any phone calls.

I wanted Chhewang back to explain to me all the things I couldn't understand and share a bowl of spicy noodles with me. I wanted to go to sleep and wake up and have it be yesterday, with another chance to get it right.

I found my satellite phone and made the call. "Jiban. Something really bad happened. Chhewang died." Speaking the words out loud made me feel like I wasn't in my body.

It was ten o'clock at night and I had woken Jiban with this horrible news. He was silent for what felt like an eternity, and then he sighed. I hated informing him like this, but I had no idea what to do. I needed help.

He began telling me it would be okay, and I shouldn't be emotional. I hadn't cried a single tear yet, and his suggestion not to be emotional made me feel guilty that I wasn't as hysterical as Pasang was. Jiban said he would send in a helicopter in the morning, and we could go look for Chhewang. He knew that Chhewang's wife, Lamu Chikee, was in a village with their boys, and he would call her. It would be okay, he said, but I knew that wasn't true. Nothing was okay.

That night, under the full moon, I lay awake in my tent. Why did this tent, one we had left at our area of Base Camp, suddenly feel so big? It had seemed so small with Chhewang and me sharing it, and now the space that he left was bigger than I could have ever imagined. I had dealt with death and accidents and the grief of others in my years of ambulance work and guiding, but I had never felt so directly entangled in it. My breath was caught in my lungs, refusing to let me exhale, so I sat awake, unable to breathe until the sun broke the horizon and another day came.

I thought the worst day of my life was behind me. Today was a new day. Still a shit day, but at least it wasn't yesterday.

But I was wrong. Today was the worst day.

The helicopter came and picked up Pasang and me, intending to take us to the accident scene to scour for any sign of Chhewang from the air. Simone Moro, the professional Italian alpinist,[*] was flying as the co-captain to one of the most experienced pilots in Nepal. The small helicopter felt unwieldy as the strong gusts of winds caused it to rise and drop. They attempted to access the valley three times before turning back, telling me over the headset that the wind was too strong and they couldn't do it. I asked if they could take us to Chhewang's village, where his wife and children had already received word of his death. We changed course, silent for the fifteen-minute flight, before touching down in the potato field outside his small house. As Pasang and I ducked out of the helicopter, I saw that the house and the front yard were filled with monks and family and that plumes of juniper were being burned in every corner. The Buddhist funeral process had already started.

We were ushered by some Sherpas I didn't know through the door of the house and into the kitchen. The house was a traditional mud-sided teahouse in a village just off the main trekking route to Everest Base Camp. I walked in through the front door, looking to the left at the small traditional dining area. It had benches with soft cushions and rugs to sit on surrounding the shiny lacquer floors that were a staple of every Sherpa teahouse. Summit certificates hung proudly on the walls along-side photos of Chhewang on the top of Everest. To my right was a dirty tapestry covering a door and behind that was the kitchen, dim with only the light of a small window casting a muted glow. The low light illumi-nated the steam rising from teacups and the smoke from the simple open-flame clay oven. A trickle of water came from the spout of a jug perched high on a wall shelf and hovered over a silver bowl, making the sound of rain on a roof. Chhewang's wife, Lamu Chikee, sat with her shoulders hunched and her dark black hair covered by a silken head-scarf, tied in the traditional way many of the Sherpa women wore it,

---

[*] This is how I met Simone. He was the only person to climb Baruntse from the side that Chhewang had avalanched down, and he knew it well. He was serious but kind to me, and I was grateful for someone who wasn't speaking only Nepali.

somewhat like a motorcycle handkerchief. She was in her mid-thirties but the grief of this reality warped her face with pain, making her appear far older. She was surrounded by a son on each side. The boys were both nearly teenagers and had solemn faces, raw with the wetness of tears they had no time to prepare for.

When I walked in, I dropped to my knees, putting my hands in the prayer position high over my head and bowing my head to the floor in a show of deep respect. Lamu Chikee's cries turned to deafening wails and drowned out the sound of my whispers: "Maf garnous. Maf garnous. Maf garnous." *I am sorry. I am sorry. I am sorry.* I felt a firm hand on my shoulder and looked up to see Ang Tshering, a friend and the cook at Camp Two on Everest. "Come here, Meli. You can't stay here. Come to my house." His house was directly across the small dirt trail from Chhewang's. He put his hand under my armpit and pulled me to my feet, dragging me out the door. My body felt heavy and my feet didn't want to move, though I wanted nothing more than to get out of there. *Why did Chhewang die and not me?* was all I could think. I deserved death far more then he had. It should have been me.

I sat in Ang Tshering's kitchen, nearly identical to Chhewang's, while he made me tea. The wails of Lamu Chikee were slowing, but I could still hear them. "You have to eat something," he said. "I make you pancakes or a sandwich, which one?" I declined, but he insisted and made me pancakes. As he mixed the flour in the bowl, he walked toward me. "It is okay. It will be okay. We are Sherpa people, and we believe the death is chosen before you are born. She is grieving and it is hard. But it is okay." I looked him in the eye, wanting the words to comfort me in a way they just wouldn't.* It wasn't okay, I wasn't okay. My heart was beating forcefully in my chest as I steeled my face against any sign of feeling. If I allowed myself to feel the heartbreak of this moment fully, it might be the opening of a door I couldn't close. I thought about my parents

---

* In a cruel continuation, I would go to his house just a few years later to console his widow after he died in an icefall avalanche on Everest.

and leaving my home as a teenager. They had worn the same protective gaze I did now. I felt cold, and I felt guilty for feeling cold. I wanted to get out of this kitchen and be alone, but I also couldn't fathom the pain of being alone and the cascade of truth that would crash down around me when I stopped holding it at a distance. There was no comfort now, not from Ang Tshering's words, or their Buddhist belief, or anything else. There was only the slow movement of time and the inescapable weight it would add to my already overloaded heart.

Over the next days I made calls to the States to explain what had happened. I replied to an email from Peter reminding me of the accident on Rainier where twelve people were killed in an icefall and he had lived. He told me he would buy me a beer when I got back to Idaho. Various Sherpas I knew visited me while I waited in a teahouse in Namche through the police investigation. They met my solemn face with solemn faces of their own. I started to understand more and more of the language, hearing the same things repeated over and over.

The tears finally came on the third day, and they didn't stop until the fifth, though the full weight of the situation remained in a distant corner of my heart, where I secured it for a future time. I still had so much to do. I couldn't use my time to consider what my future would hold and what I would do next beyond trying to find Chhewang. The Sherpa family I stayed with welcomed me into their prayer room daily and reinforced the words Ang Tshering had said on the first day—it was all as it should be. I met one of Chhewang's little brothers and sat in silence as he wailed when I handed him Chhewang's cell phone.

On the fifth day we took a flight, again with Simone and Pasang, attempting to find any sign of Chhewang. We were able to get close to the face of the mountain, but not high enough with the weight of all the passengers, so the captain landed in a vacant field and asked me and Chhewang's brother to get out. The helicopter took off over our heads, leaving us in a cloud of dust, silence, and tremendous discomfort. I thought about the comfortable silence I had with Chhewang and my chest squeezed tight against my heart, aching. Chhewang's brother wished he hadn't met me. He wished I didn't exist. I could see it in his face. I, too, wished I didn't exist. I imagined the roles being reversed and Chhewang standing next to my sister. "I want to do whatever I can," I said slowly, in a whisper. "For the family, I mean. He was a friend to me. I want to do whatever I can." There were no words to convey what I wanted to say. Words couldn't convey the expanse of regret and guilt I was feeling. I had survived. He hadn't.

His brother looked at me with sharp eyes but said no words. The *whoomph* of the helicopter filled the silence again as it landed to retrieve us. There was no sign of him. Just huge avalanches. Just vast space. Just the heavy ice hanging precariously above a jumble of avalanche debris. There was no chance, Simone said. Not any chance.

* * *

A few days later, after signing a police report written entirely in Nepali and translated by someone I just had to trust, I was allowed to fly back to Kathmandu. I went to the pharmacy and got a packet of Ambien to force the sleep I knew I couldn't find on my own. I had meetings with the Ministry of Tourism and the insurance agent who would pay Chhewang's wife his life insurance. The CEO of Eddie Bauer contacted me to send condolences and let me know he wanted to pay the helicopter bills. They were nearing $19,000, and I hadn't thought about how I would pay them, but of course they would be my bills. Chhewang hadn't had rescue insurance and even if he had, the private hiring of a helicopter to fly at those high altitudes wouldn't be covered. The bill was mine. A group of Sherpas decided they wanted to do an expedition on foot to find Chhewang. They believed he might still be alive somehow and they needed to go get him. It had been ten days since the accident. Whatever remained of my heart shattered into a million pieces as I imagined the group of five wandering on the dangerous route with avalanches all around. What if they died? "Please don't go!" I begged Tshering Dorje. He had summited Everest on my first trip and been our Sirdar the previous spring when Dave Morton and I had gone up in my failed attempt to summit without oxygen. I couldn't face the possibility of his two daughters being fatherless alongside Chhewang's sons. I couldn't do it again. I couldn't endure any more tragedy.

"Sorry, Didi. We go." He said this simply as we stood in the safe and comfortable lobby of the hotel. "You pay for the life insurance, okay?" He didn't ask as much as tell me what I had to do. There were very few choices left for me now. I agreed, not because I wanted to, but because I was becoming all too familiar with the forced choices you make when the world careens out of control in front of you. Back in my hotel room, the phone rang, and I answered, wondering what anger might be there for me.* It was Ian. He was back from his river trip, and he had heard, through the Sherpa-net,† what had happened. He said he was tired and worn down after almost a month of living on the river and teaching and training young Nepalis to be river guides. But he could meet me for lunch. I hadn't eaten much more than crackers and gummy bears since I got back to Kathmandu, and I thought seeing him might be nice. I wanted to tell the story to someone who spoke English. I needed to get it all out in a way I hadn't yet.

I met him a few hours later at a touristy Italian restaurant in Kathmandu. Over a hot plate of lasagna, I told him what had happened. He nodded and listened, and I felt grateful just to talk. As I ended my rambling about what was next, he set his fork down and leaned back on his chair, crossing his arms defensively over his chest.

"What's wrong?" I asked, sensing something was coming. In his soft and seductive Scottish accent, he said, "I have just had a shit past

---

* It wasn't anger, but it felt like it in those days. Each Sherpa who asked me to tell the story of what happened seemed angry. I had taken something from them. I had a kind of shame that made every interaction feel like a guilty one. And it would take years to work through that and create enough space to see that pain and anger are mirrors of each other in grief of loss.

† The fastest mode of information exchange known to man.

month." I hadn't even asked. He continued, his soft accent gaining a harder edge. "And you know what? On expeditions, people die. It wasn't your fault." He said this so assertively. "You weren't even there, it's not like you cut the rope." His practicality stung, though I suspected he was actually trying to help. He had been through many harrowing experiences that were far worse than this, he reassured me. I would be fine. But instead of comfort, his words were a smack in the face, bringing me to the present moment and all the pain it contained. I looked at him with disgust. I was hoping he would hold my broken heart, but instead he had told me to stop my whining. I hated him in that moment and couldn't wait to put more space between us.

I paid for my lunch and walked the dusty street back to my hotel as he took a motorbike back to his. The next day, I was told I could finally go home. I changed my flight for the third time and made my way to the airport. Waves of nausea accompanied me on the twenty hours of flying. I touched down in the U.S., sure that every person who saw me could tell what had happened. I was so used to being greeted with the assignment of "You were with Chhewang Nima" that I expected the customs officer to know it too. But he didn't. I was anonymous again.

My bags were lost somewhere in India, and I had a layover in Seattle. I went to my friend Christine's house to be near someone who knew me, someone who knew how flawed I was and chose to love me anyway. I had met Christine five years earlier while we were both working for a remote medical company, and she had allowed me into her life right when her mother died, sharing a vulnerability that I admired. Christine always opened her couch to me and never made me feel bad for not calling unless I needed something. She was one of the only girlfriends I had managed to keep for more than a year at a time, and I knew she could hold some of my grief while expecting nothing from me. I was just floating in the ocean, bobbing along in the calm waves and rough seas, equally out of control in either. I greeted Christine and quickly hid in her dark bedroom with the curtains drawn. I wanted to be near her but alone. I was starting to consider what my life was going to look like next.

Could I go back to climbing? Could I ever return to Nepal? I wasn't who I thought I was going to be, and now really bad things were happening. People were dying. It was no longer just a broken family or a broken heart. It was far bigger than that.

As afternoon turned to evening, sharp pains shot like lightning bolts from my abdomen down my legs. The nausea from the flight hadn't gone away. I felt like I was being broken open from the inside out. I felt like everything was coming in waves. I would get to feel okay just long enough for the next wave of electric pain to crash over me in a surprise, even though I expected it.

Christine insisted I see a doctor. I didn't have the energy to resist, so I climbed into my rental car and navigated to an urgent care clinic a few miles from her house.* The clinic staff greeted my arrival with concern; I must have looked like the death with which I seemed to be keeping company. I gave a nurse my medical history and my blood and waited for a doctor. He came in, holding a clipboard and a folder, a serious look on his face. "Can I ask you . . . did you know that you were pregnant?"

No hello. No "I'm Dr. So-and So . . ."

No, I did not know that. I flashed on the one-night stand that Ian and I had shared in Kathmandu. I still took birth control pills, so none of this made any sense. What was happening? The world narrowed around me. All the doctor's words sounded muffled with cotton. Ultrasound, not viable, low blood pressure, give fluid, miscarriage. My body was rejecting life. Everything around me was dying. Everything inside me, too. I rode the waves of information and took the medicine and

---

* As I crossed the interstate at my exit, the car in front of me abruptly slammed on their brakes, causing me to do the same and sending the car behind me smack into me in a jarring crush of crunching metal. I limped my broken self from my broken rental car to the side of the road and waited for the cops and tow trucks to come. Everyone was fine, just property damage. I remembered my dad telling me catastrophe travels in threes and I wondered what might be next. This didn't feel like real life.

called Christine to come and get me. She met me in the lobby and said, "You have got to be fucking kidding me."

I started laughing. It felt inappropriate and good. "Nope. I can't make this up." My laughter turned to exhausted tears as she drove me to her house, as she tucked me into bed. Tomorrow would be better, she promised.

I lay awake, googling the time zone in Bhutan, where Ian was now. I felt like I should tell him. Not that it mattered, but I just thought he should know. When it was ten a.m. there, I dialed his number and caught him, to my surprise. My voice felt weak as I tried to summon the courage to just speak the truth. "I told you I wasn't feeling well. I went to the doctor . . ." He offered an *uh-huh* and a *mm-hmm* as I spoke, making me wonder if he was doing something else while we talked. "I am, well, I was pregnant, I guess. It was a miscarriage." I swallowed my own words, making them come out in a near whisper. I didn't want to talk or think about this. But he met my words with silence and I couldn't deal with any more silence, either, so I ushered him off the phone by telling him I needed to go. He said it was probably all for the best, as he didn't want kids, as I knew. I agreed and hung up, throwing my phone across the room.

Catastrophe comes in threes. Now I had the full set. No more. I fell into a groggy medication-induced sleep and woke the next morning for my flight home. My bags were still in India, but I was going to be in my own space, alone. I couldn't wait.

Once I got there, I showered and put on my coziest clothes and stayed in them, in the dark of my condo, for the next two weeks. I hung blankets over the windows and left only once to get food, going late at night to avoid seeing anyone I knew. I texted with Christine and floated the idea of moving away from Sun Valley. I didn't have anything important there anyway. She encouraged me to not make any rushed decisions. I agreed but wanted to take a trip to Colorado anyway, just to see how it felt. I would go see my parents, not for comfort as much as for a reminder that I could survive hard things. It was what I did when my life fell apart. It was the scab I would pick off to see that I could bleed and heal again. I was resilient and I would be okay, and seeing them would prove that.

As I drove on the open highway through Utah, I saw the full moon rising. It had been one month. Chhewang died on a full moon. And now the moon was full again. Time didn't care that his boys didn't have a dad. Time didn't care that I felt empty and unattached to everything that used to ground me. Feeling unattached allowed me to avoid the deep hurt of everything that was happening in my life. The emptiness was better than feeling the oppressive pain, though it was painful in its own way. But there was no pause for my pain. Chhewang had died, and I had faced his family and then faced Ian. I had returned home and lost a part of myself. I had cried and stopped crying, and I had imagined what it would feel like for time to stop, freezing me here in this pain. But time just kept going. The full moon would wane and then come back again whether I was hurt or healed.

I cried deep, wet tears from my heart. I woke up from bad dreams far more often than I wanted to admit, and so I quieted the trauma, telling myself that I was in fact lucky. I just needed to move on. If the moon could keep going, couldn't I? What was the alternative? If I stopped everything, it would always be this way. If I left Sun Valley, I would always remember it in the light of this pain. If I never put my crampons back on, I would never get a chance to know the beauty of the mountains; I would be left with only the despair. The moon wasn't going to stop for my pain. The sliver of self I had left with could return to wholeness, fullness, again. I was alive, and now I had to live. But I had to go back to Nepal. I had to face Chhewang's wife and his boys again and sit with all that they had lost. And now that I was broken open, I had to finally face myself. There was no other choice.

IV

13.

NO PICKET FENCE

2012: Everest, Nepal

The year that followed Baruntse and the accident was one of contradictions. My heart was broken in a way I couldn't have imagined. The pain felt searing and unending, reminding me of what it was like to be a teenager. But it wasn't a pain I could simply outgrow. It would require doing things differently than I ever had. Up to this point, I had been swimming along the surface of my life with my head above water so I would never have to look at the darkness I was holding below. I was moving in and out of relationships with men, primarily using them for what they had that I wanted. I was avoiding deep friendships out of fear that I would have to show myself to someone and they might not love what they saw. And I was filling my days with running away disguised as adventure. If I had another mountain to climb, I wouldn't have to sit still long enough to face where I was. For my life to truly begin to change I knew that it would require me to hold open the broken parts and let them get some air—just to see if they could heal.

Knowing this, though, was not the same as doing it. And so I returned to the mountains, an escape that had become well practiced. I climbed uphill and over glaciers. I passed under rockfall and icefall and tiptoed past avalanche paths. I tried to get to the summit of Everest again, but turned back, willing to retreat without the summit in exchange for the lessons that being at altitude for months could teach me. I set intentions for how my life would be now. There had been so many "before and after" moments in my life, and this was another one, though different from the others in many ways. I grew quickly into someone who wore the weathered lines of tragedy on her face. But I kept climbing. And I kept living, feeling it was the only choice I had, after being surrounded by Chhewang's death. I wanted not just to live, but to live and be a good person. I felt like maybe I deserved this tragedy on some level because of all I had done wrong. I felt guilty that Chhewang had died and I had lived. In the months after his death, I was paralyzed by the thoughts of what his family was enduring; somehow it all felt like my fault. I revisited the debate about whether I should just stop climbing, wondering if that would fix any of this, but knowing that it wouldn't.

For the past nine years I had absorbed myself into the mountains, and mostly they had welcomed me. Somewhere in between the summits and the failures, the mountains had slowly and surely become who I was at my core. It was what defined me; I was a mountain climber. It was something I had wanted so badly years ago, to be someone who was adventurous and persistent. And in many ways, that is who I had always been, but the mountains had allowed me a place to display my tenacity and curiosity on a stage that the world looked up to instead of down on. The escape wasn't seen as running away; it was seen as truly living. And it felt good.

I was so well practiced at escaping. But I was also starting to see that what I was really trying to outrun was so deep inside me that mountains wouldn't free me. I wanted to accept that what I needed wasn't going to be found somewhere else. I had to stop exchanging one discomfort for another, discarding my life experiences like clothes that no longer fit, and stay in the outfit I chose. It wasn't about running away; it was about turning and facing what was, and trying, for once, to accept it.

When Jon had arrived in my life—strong-jawed, tall, athletic, confident but not cocky—I was broken in so many ways. He showed up with genuine curiosity about who I was and a tenderness that I needed. And he was persistent. I pushed him away for weeks as I wrapped myself in both grief and recovery, but he continued to gently show up, offering a little spot of sweetness in a very bitter time. I was uniquely vulnerable, far more than I had been in the years past, and through that little crack in my tough exterior, his love and care seeped in. When I thought about us being together, it felt like a fairy tale. The hockey player and the mountain climber. He had a soft innocence to him, the mark of a life unburdened with childhood traumas. I wondered if he would truly accept me with all my baggage, and in many ways, I felt undeserving of his attention. He reminded me of the clean-cut, well-educated athlete that the popular girls in high school dated. I didn't date those guys, or rather, they didn't date me. I carried too many wounds on my sleeve, and my story wasn't going to be a fairy tale. I wasn't a cheerleader to any quarterback.

But Jon didn't know any of that when we met. And so as we dated and began to fall in love, I committed to opening myself up as completely as I could. I softened my exterior and held his hand at dinner, cuddling against him in public, not afraid of being seen as something other than completely independent. I watched movies with him and spent my time trying to truly know him as I let him in on my biggest fears and didn't try to explain away why it was all fine. I sat in silence with him, and I put him first in my thoughts and actions.

It was terrifying. I had still-raw wounds from my preteen years. To let someone in required that I opened the weeping abrasions on my heart to the cold and stinging wind of vulnerability. This was a foreign language, but I was committed to becoming fluent. To do so would mean quieting the part of me that reveled in being impenetrable and unhurtable, the me who practiced keeping everyone at two arms' length because one was never enough.

I went to each of Jon's hockey games in our early days of dating, standing with the other wives and girlfriends, attempting to connect. I felt extremely out of my element but I knew that I had to push myself for things to be different. Jon would see me as he skated off the ice at breaks and he would nod his strong jaw lovingly in my direction, a little *Thank you, I see you.* After the games, we would go to dinner with the team and then spend hours lying in bed, talking. He came from a big family, with three boys and a girl. His father was a high-performing attorney who had instilled the importance of education and curiosity in all the kids. His mom was a loving caretaker, doing everything she could to make sure her kids felt loved. Jon was smart, and well-educated. He went to a private college on the East Coast and quickly rose to the top of any role he took on. He worked as a journalist and then moved into nonprofit community management, with an eye on local government someday. We would talk about things big and small. We would discuss the deeper meaning behind Banksy's work and debate politics. He challenged my views and showed me completely new ones. And he was funny. He had a kind of sarcasm that reminded me of my father's humor. I told him about my childhood and how helpless I had felt. He held me close, unable to relate because of his own near-perfect upbringing, but he listened, and that was enough. I was smitten. He was, too.

On our first Christmas together, I created a scavenger hunt with little poems and notes, leading him all over town and ending with a soak in a natural hot spring that was carefully dammed next to the cold winter river in Idaho. "I didn't know what to give you. So I am giving you this." I handed him the final gift—it was a small box with a tiny paper inside, and a cut-out heart. "I love you." I said the words back to him, and for the first time in my life it wasn't with the intention of getting something. It was true. It was how I felt. I didn't want his life or what he had. I just wanted his love, and I was going to have to start by giving him mine.

"I want to be with you forever." He whispered the words through gentle kisses. I told him he had to wait four seasons to decide if he could. I was a different person when the seasons changed, I warned. I would try to run away. I would put the mountain first. He promised this wouldn't scare him, and one year later, after our fourth season together, he proposed to me in another beautiful Idaho hot spring. I said yes, without any fear of what might be ahead.

If up to that point I felt I hadn't been good at all, now I intended to be good in that wholesome, white-picket-fence, middle-America way. The way Jon's brother's wives were. I would blend in and become one of them. It was my intent to be the good wife to the good husband. To be a real couple. To have our windows be the ones anyone could easily look into while walking a dog after dusk; nothing to hide in our house.

But I had never lived in a house with windows for people to see into. I had never lived without a dark hidden truth that only I knew—the truth of my not-goodness. Thinking that I could somehow just decide finally to be good, and then it would simply happen, was like deciding I was going to speak Mandarin and opening my mouth only to have familiar English tumble out. I had decided so many things in my life that I was able to make happen. I decided to become a mountain climber, I decided to climb Everest, I decided to leave my parents' home at seventeen and support myself. But this was different. This was deciding what to *be,* not what to do. Doing something, and the action that propelled me forward, felt like movement. But deciding who to be wasn't about action at all. That was about clarifying the character underneath the action, something I had avoided doing for a very long time. But I couldn't see that clearly, and I expected that if I decided I could be all the things I wanted to be, I would somehow make it happen.

I didn't let Jon know how much it took out of me to open myself emotionally. I spent all my time analyzing my every action in our relationship, and berating myself anytime I felt I got it wrong. It was a laborious dance of deciding what to do, trying to do it, and then reviewing all the ways I could have done it better. Living that way was exhausting. I would cry in the shower and then steel myself and try again to be better. I lavished Jon with love and gratitude and affection, things that were so hard for me. I didn't look at him as a tool for my work, but instead as another person, complex and imperfect but willing to do this life with me. I was excited for our lives together. I was excited to have a true partner and a safe place—a place where I didn't have to always be strong and resilient.

But excitement about a thing is only one ingredient. I had a big mountain to climb to be ready for partnership, and I knew it. I couldn't just wish things would shift; I had to work toward the change. I had spent the previous years building walls around my heart and keeping my partners at a distance. It felt necessary to avoid heartache, but it had repeatedly ended poorly. I wanted this to be different.

The effort it took me to be fully present and vulnerable with Jon made my annual work pilgrimage to Everest* feel like a welcome break. As the spring, and my departure, got closer, I noticed that I was less patient with Jon's curiosity about my life on the mountain. "Do you just sleep in one tent at high camp, all of you in an orgy?" he asked with sarcasm. I bristled at his joke and lack of knowledge of the place I felt most at home, but then I immediately felt guilty for judging him. Why would he know? So instead, I would explain the details and remind him that it would be him that I would be thinking of while I was away. And when I returned, we would get married. But when I was away on the

---

* Jon was not a climber at all. I used to joke and say I was way smarter than to marry a climber when people asked if my husband climbed too. He wanted to learn about it, but his main athletic love was hockey. He came from a family of hockey players and he had skated that path as well. Walking uphill slowly was not his thing, and so it got to remain solely my thing.

mountain, I no longer had to hold open my steel outer armor. And after even a short time together, it wasn't letting my guard down that felt good—it was putting it back up.

* * *

It was spring of 2012, and I was migrating back to Everest, this time to guide a cameraman to the summit as he captured the journey of Peter's cousin, Leif Whittaker, the son of the first American to summit Everest, Jim Whittaker. The cameraman, Kent Harvey, was a friend, and we had shared many tents together on many mountains, including on Everest in 2009. On that trip everyone had affectionately called Kent, then in his early forties, Old Man Harvey, because he had the worry and hunch of a much older, wearier soul. I found his anxiety pleasant to be around—he unconsciously put to words the fears that everyone had but was too proud to say.

I was less thrilled about working with Dave Hahn. Our history was complicated. Dave had been someone I looked up to in my first days of guiding. He was the summitingest* non-Sherpa Everest climber, with fifteen, and he had what seemed like a thousand years of experience guiding around the world. In Alaska and on Rainier he was clever and humble, sharing tales of Everest climbs and near-fatal poo tent incidents at Base Camp in a slow, hypnotizing cadence. Sometimes he fell into an unnaturally long pause midstory, as if his inner computer's cursor was stuck pinwheeling. And yet just as I was questioning if the high altitude had finally gotten to him, a moment later—BAM! He would come out with the sharpest, most quick-witted thing you'd ever heard. He was over six feet tall with size-fifteen feet, a combination that made him seem like a giraffe with rabbit feet, and just as awkward. But somehow he could traipse gracefully over jagged rocky and icy terrain with the precision of a lynx.

---

* Is that a thing? It should be a thing.

Dave had featured in both my worst and my best days of guiding during my first year working on Rainier. The worst came at the culmination of hard climbs made harder by the torrent of minimization and sexualization from male clients. I had just come off a climb in which the leader of a nine-man group from Utah gestured to me and said to the lead guide, "We don't want to tie into the rope with *her*. With a girl. A small girl. I mean, what would we tell our wives? Can she even carry the rope?" My very next climb was with Dave, and it was the same story—jokes about girls, jokes about me, feeling simultaneously ogled and marginalized. I tried to stand taller and profess my skills more forcefully, but it failed.* When I got down after wasting two days of my life, I stomped into Peter's office and quit. He and the owners, probably loath to reschedule the whole season without me, tried to convince me to ride it out. For my next scheduled climb, the father/daughter clients had requested a female guide, and I was the only one available. But Dave Hahn was leading it. After an agonizing moment of uncertainty, I swallowed my discontent and resigned to stay.

That climb turned out to be the best experience of my first season. Dave was night and day from the previous climb; kindness had replaced his condescension. He took me under his wing and showed me how to do things more efficiently. He let me lead our rope team of four out onto the glacier, exploring a crisscross path through the crevasses to show the clients the deep internal walls of the glacier's voids. He told me stories of working on Everest and shared secrets of how to move efficiently on fixed lines. I felt valued.

Over the years, my relationship with Dave played out across the polarities of those first-year climbs: a pendulum swing between feeling powerful and powerless. On my first climb of Everest, he was there guiding, and had helped quell my anxiety when it peaked before the summit

---

* The funny thing about wanting respect in that environment, and most environments, is the more you assert all the reasons you deserve the respect, the further away it gets. But ego is a curtain you cannot see that truth through.

push. But later in 2009, he openly questioned my capability to climb Everest with Ed Viesturs as my partner. He spoke over me and he spoke for me. His humility at lower elevations swelled into an ego that was impenetrable when he was on Everest.

So, in 2012, when Eddie Bauer put us together for another expedition, I was both thrilled for the work and hesitant to rejoin Dave. But my desire to be on Everest again trumped my concern. Plus, I would have Kent with me, a brother in arms. Kent and I would joke that we were part of a Russian regime; I would call him Boris and he would call me Tatiana. And I would be silently subversive to the system of power that I didn't feel like I belonged in. I hung a simple white sheet of paper on the wall of our dining tent with an Abraham Lincoln quote written in Sharpie: "Nearly all men can stand adversity, but if you want to test a man's character, give him power."

The season was moving forward with the expected rhythm of a team finding their balance together until suddenly everything went upside down. The genesis of the tension was a simple question: "Dave, do you train for the Everest season? I mean, outside of work?" I asked him over breakfast. I had really committed to training that previous winter, and I suddenly felt curious if he did anything or just relied on his experience and annual work to keep him strong. He looked at me squarely. He had not heard the curiosity I was expressing, but rather someone questioning his fitness. Our entire team would be punished for my question.

From that day forward Dave set out on any day hike, or climb, at a blazing speed. Leif could mostly keep up, but Kent and I never could. This led to tense discussions in the tent between Dave and me. "Take a walk, Melissa." He spoke firmly as he leaned forward. "You can decide if you really want to be here. I think you are pissed that *you* aren't the leader, but you need to accept that I am. If you can, then you can stay."*

---

* I am now sure that my ego was annoyed at minimum and openly bleeding at maximum at my role as an assistant, but I think Dave also had that under a microscope, making it seem much bigger than it was.

When I gave input on our plan, it felt like he always did the opposite and that we were for some reason engaged in a war. I wanted to stay, so I took the walk and swallowed my frustrations.

All of this swirled in me along with my other engagement, to Jon. The last time I'd worked with Dave, in 2009, he had seen the demise of my engagement to Ian. I wondered if Dave was anticipating the same outcome now. But I wanted to be seen as a different person, someone who had grown through the pain of the previous years. I wouldn't back out of my engagement this time. This time was different.

But in the weeks preceding my departure for Nepal I had begun to feel the quiet breath of longing for freedom and aloneness, and yearning for my protective guard. I tried to extinguish those thoughts, ignore them, and not allow them to grow. But a seed of doubt can grow a noxious weed, spreading dominantly no matter how you try to remove it. Once it is there, its roots will work their way into the ground and force their way up everywhere.

On the expedition, I tried to keep the doubt away by writing to Jon in the little green journal we shared. I called him on the sat phone almost every day. I wore a silver band on my left hand in place of the engagement ring I left at home, a clear sign to all those lonely expedition men that I was taken and not for the taking. I talked about Jon, extending my vulnerability to sharing things about my personal life with the people who I previously valued seeing me as independent, solo. Trying to stay committed to my relationship and future was so hard in this place where relationships were transient. I had practiced keeping on-guard over the years, and now trying to stay open felt awkward and uneasy. Paired with the dismissiveness I was experiencing on this expedition, it became the perfect solvent to break down all my trying to be "good."

And now, midway through the season, it was clear to me that it was no use. The grip I had on the life I was trying to live was slipping with each moment. Deciding that I could be healed by ignoring all the parts of myself that were jagged and sharp wasn't the same as deciding to climb a mountain. I couldn't brute-force my way into being someone I wasn't. I wasn't good. It was just an act. The seed of doubt about my ability to stay vulnerable was growing and propagating into an unruly field—vast and expansive, overtaking all the work I had done to keep it away. I was starting to wonder if it was better to be alone and at ease than to work so relentlessly at being a good partner. Selfishness had a certain shiny allure, and it was drawing me further in. This life in the mountains was so innately selfish—the pursuit of a summit stance for a moment benefits only the person who stands there. And that practice of self-focused living was starting to feel like the only way I could live.

The expedition, in terms of getting Leif to the summit, was a success. Everyone fulfilled their role and did their job. I summited for my fourth time, Dave for his sixteenth. We had formed an unspoken truce enough to get on with the task at hand and complete the job.

The season had unfolded without more than the common drama of any year, but somehow it also ended with me feeling far worse than I had at the start. I felt a restless discontent continuing to grow inside me. At the end of the expedition, desperate for some space, I chose to walk out of Base Camp with the Nepali staff, a day ahead of Dave and the rest of the team. They would walk all twenty-six miles (which I was splitting into two days) in one day, and then we would reunite on the trail for our shared flight out. That was the plan.

Two days later, when I reached the teahouse that was meant to be our meeting location, I could see immediately that no one from my team was there, just another guide asking questions. "I bet you're pissed about your team!" he said to me as I walked in.

I didn't know how he could know that I had been existing separately from my team for nearly the entire expedition, so I played it cool. "Why?" I asked. My naivete must have seemed both quaint and sad. All I had wanted was to be included, to be valued. And here I was, wondering what this person knew about my team that I did not.

But he wasn't talking about my role within my team. He was talking about what had happened since I left. "They flew out of Base Camp on a helicopter right after you started walking yesterday. They are already back in Kathmandu."

My blood boiled and my stomach knotted. *Those motherfuckers.* Of course they did. Dave had never wanted me to be part of the expedition, and even though Kent had been my main friend for the past forty days, his loyalty stayed with our leader. No matter how much time I spent on this mountain, I would never be able to enter the boys' club.

I began angrily pulling together the logistics of getting my own helicopter back to Kathmandu the next morning, sharing it with a team that wasn't mine but was happy to include me. When I arrived back at the hotel by taxi, I got out to see Kent, my unfaithful Boris, sitting on the marble steps outside with an "Oh, shit" look on his face. "I tried to call you. I'm sorry, Tatiana."

He was clean and showered and laundered. I was dusty, hungry, and pissed. With a hushed tone, he said, "We are going to lunch right now." His body was turned slightly away from me, as though he was unsure if I would hit or hug him. I couldn't go to lunch without a shower. I was wearing the stench of the summit push and the dust of a trail none of them had even walked.

Dave came out to the marble steps, clearly surprised to see me. "Oh, hey," he said, ever the awkward giraffe. "We are going to lunch, if you want to come." He didn't expect me to come; I could see that in the way he offered while half starting to walk away.

"Okay, I'm coming," I said, setting my dirty backpack filled with dirty things down on my pile of duffel bags, knowing it would wait for me in the lobby until I returned. Rage bubbled inside me as we ate in silence, not addressing the elephant in the room.

Back at the hotel, I showered, drank all the beer in the minibar, and reveled in my clean clothes. I shaved my legs and blow-dried my sun-bleached blond hair. My body was thin, and I didn't fit into my clothes in the way I had before the sixty days of high-altitude atrophy. I slipped into a black skirt and a white shirt with a Nepali scarf wrapped around my neck. It felt good to feel pretty. On the mountain I wanted to be the same as all the men, but at sea level I wanted to be different.

I should have called Jon. I should have stayed in. Instead, I texted another climber who I knew was in Kathmandu, someone who wasn't part of my team or my drama, asking to meet for drinks after dinner. I didn't need the boys on my team who never included me. I would eat with them and then leave them behind. I wanted to feel wanted and then leave, no vulnerability required. I wanted to break the foundation I had built with Jon—it wasn't something I ever deserved in the first place.

It could have been my anger at not feeling valued or the comfort of not having to be vulnerable. Or just the erosive power of distance that led me to water the seeds of doubt about my ability to be with Jon. I didn't doubt him, but rather myself. It was so much easier to be who I had always been than to grow into someone new. I just wanted to escape from the vulnerability I had agreed to maintain. But I couldn't just leave. I couldn't call off another wedding. I was stuck, needing to stay but also needing to escape.

So at the end of the text to my friend asking to meet up, I included the kiss-blowing emoji—an invitation I knew would be understood. And I didn't care. I wanted something simple, something that didn't require work. I wanted to feel something. I wanted to feel needed in a primal and impermanent way. It is easier to be the one who destroys things than to be destroyed. It is easier to run away than to find out that you are not lovable even when you are trying so hard to be good.

My flirting texts turned into a flirting dinner and flirting drinks. The drinks turned to sneaking down an alley, away from the group, and slipping into a taxi headed for a hotel that wasn't either of ours. The hotel turned into a night of forgetting about Dave Hahn and how he didn't value me.* Forgetting about Jon and how he did. And in the morning, I

---

* Apparently, I am kind of still pissed at Dave Hahn, which comes as a bit of a surprise. I thought I didn't care. But it should be noted that I don't blame him for my slippery behavior. That was all me, and I likely would have done it anyway, even if the season had been perfect.

exited the hotel, a person with a secret and a whole garden of doubt at what my life even was anymore.

I knew I would never tell Jon. He flew from Idaho to Thailand to meet me at the end of the season, a sort of pre-wedding honeymoon, since I would spend the summer working right after our actual wedding. In Thailand, we took a small boat to a little island in a torrential rainstorm. The beach was absconded by the high tide of a major monsoonal storm, and it felt appropriate. "You seem like you're somewhere else," Jon said to me gently as I stiffened with the slightest touch of his hand.

"It's just the end-of-the-season transition. It is hard. It's part of it. If you don't like it, maybe you should go home." I antagonized him with my brooding words, hoping he would just go.

But he didn't. He stayed the course and his lovingness hurt, knowing that I had already broken my promise to be faithful. I just had to get through this and then the next thing and maybe I could pretend none of this had happened. We ended the honeymoon with me holding him at a distance, and him accepting this as part of being with someone who lived half their life away on expeditions. I knew I would go home and pretend that everything was fine and he would willingly accept it, wanting to believe that things were.

We returned to our house and the intense lush green of spring, a contrast to the lack of life in the high mountains. Jon's family arrived to spend time with us in the weeks before the wedding and I quickly busied myself with getting things ready, ignoring my guilt and trying again to be the woman he thought he was marrying. I would crush the knowledge that I wasn't ready to be married and I would dress it in white and decorate my doubt with flowers. I would stand in front of all our friends and promise to be faithful and open and do this journey together. I would look at myself in the mirror and know that a liar was looking back—someone who didn't even know themselves, and someone who didn't even want to.

14.

THINNER THAN AIR

2013: Everest, Nepal

My body ached with the yearning for the simple pleasure of oxygen and sleep. I twisted around, a marshmallow stuffed in a marshmallow, my down suit twisting up into my sleeping bag with each small movement. The little green glow of my watch said 3:40 a.m. The sun would be coming up in a few hours and we could get the hell out of here.

The South Col, at 26,000 feet, was no place to linger. The tent was flapping loudly in the relentless wind as Tshering Dorje and I nestled against each other unintentionally on the uneven rocks that constituted the tent platform. One name, over and over, kept running through my head on vicious repeat. I wanted sleep. I wanted a new word in my head. I wanted out of this loop I was stuck in. But no.

Alexey Bolotov. Alexey Bolotov. Alexey Bolotov. Alexey Bolotov.

The only thought in my mind was the name of a person I barely knew. Senseless. Confusing. Appropriate, though, after a season that had been marked by those feelings the entire time. How had this place that was so sacred and so infinite come to feel so scarred and confining? The mountain that had been my classroom for so many years was suddenly a dark maze with dead ends at every turn. That was the lesson. That was the way. Stop, stay where you are. Be still. Learn about all the contours of the discomfort you are in instead of trying to exchange it for something new. *Alexey Bolotov. Alexey Bolotov. Alexey Bolotov.*

Two months ago, at home, in the final days of packing for my now annual Everest expedition, I had begun to feel the familiar and frenetic energy of being ready to leave. It had become my habit each spring to begin a calculated and rigorous distancing practice from the comforts of my life in the weeks prior to my departure. If I separated myself emotionally from the people and the comforts, I convinced myself, I would be more acclimated to the distance when the time came to fly across the globe and exist with limited communication or closeness for sixty days. But I also knew there was something comforting about the distance. I still reveled in the aloneness. It was my own private space and there was only room for one in there.

This season, though, was going to be different. One night after too many beers at a bar in Idaho, I had decided to invite a small group of friends from home to join me on the trek into Base Camp. I would share with them this special world that felt more like home to me than our small Idaho town ever would. Instead of aloneness I would embrace the togetherness. And I would bring Jon. My husband of one year.* They would be my send-off crew, and they would attend a second marriage ceremony for Jon and me. This one would be hosted by the Sherpa fam-

---

* And what a fucking year. I entered a dark slump following the wedding. The closer I looked at our union, and at him, the more I wondered if I had married him solely so that I could be someone's wife, instead of marrying him for who he truly was. And I wondered if he had married the media's version of me—"badass mountaineer." I was cocktail-party conversation for him more than a person to share a life with. We were playing the part in each other's stories, but we weren't ever in the same one.

ily I was closest with and be in the Sherpa tradition. It seemed like a good idea, if I didn't think too much about it.

But as I had packed the final items for my long expedition and noticed that Jon's duffel bag was nearly as big as mine, a sort of suffocating feeling took over. I had kept my worlds separate, existing in duality but never in unison. And now I was going to let my two existences overlap. Why was I doing this? What good could come from exposing my private place, and the person I was in that place, to my new husband? My mountain self felt like the truest version of me, but what if my new husband didn't like the me that I loved the most? I felt afraid in a way I hadn't since I was young. I was carrying the guilt that I had been unfaithful and the fear that he might somehow find out. And I was nestling all that inside the idea that even if he never did find out, I would still know. I wasn't who I was pretending to be.

My fear was muted by the familiarity of a place I loved so much. I showed my friends and Jon the trail, and the places with the spiciest curry. I showed them me, in silence, a person they had rarely seen. On the third day we arrived at the home of my closest Sherpa family and we were greeted by Cherap, as warm and loving as my own father.* He prepared Jon and the boys for the Sherpa wedding ceremony as all the elder Sherpani prepared me and my girlfriends.

"Come here, Jon, we will show you how Sherpa do this." Cherap was generous with his knowledge as he led Jon to a room with the other Sherpa men and our male friends. Jon was almost a foot taller than Cherap, and he stood proud with his shoulders squared and back in contrast to Cherap's humble, easeful slouch.

"Is this the bachelor party?" Jon said in jest, making good-natured jokes in his discomfort.

"This is the Zendi, the final wedding. In our culture this is the

---

* Cherap had taken me in after Chhewang died and treated me with the love he showed everyone. He taught me about Sherpa traditions and shared stories of his young life. I loved him and his wife, Lhakpa Doma, and all the love they gave to me.

union of not two people, but two families," Cherap explained slowly. "From this day forward, your wife will live now with your parents and take care of them. We will act as her parents in the ceremony, giving her to your family." As Cherap explained the ritual, the group's elder Sherpas helped Jon into a yak's-wool-lined robe and elaborate brimmed hat reminiscent of a cowboy hat.

"I don't know if you can give Melissa away. She belongs to no one," Jon said with a laugh. But under the joke and the smirk was the seed of truth that he already knew. I imagined that he had felt me put distance between us even as we prepared for this cultural celebration of our union. He had spent two years in the push-pull of my attempts to keep close while slowly tiptoeing away. He was smart. But he was also in love, and love can be the glare of the sun in your eyes, preventing you from seeing things as they are.

The girls gathered in another area, where we learned that all the women must wear braids. We donned traditional Sherpani dresses, with the married women getting an apron and the single women going without one. We were told that as soon as the ceremony was complete, it would be the job of all the married women (including me) to circle the room and serve food to the attendees. I could do that. It was also the duty of the bride to cry during the ceremony, as after this she would leave her family to go live forever with her husband's family. I couldn't do that. I was never a big crier to begin with, and crying on command usually resulted in church giggles that became uncontrollable. But I would do my best. It was how I had gotten through the year behind me, by just trying to keep moving and do what was expected of me.

The ceremony was beautifully calm and gave way to raucous dancing, drinking, and laughing, in true Sherpa style. We sat in front of a Lama who read Tibetan scripts and blessed our union. Rhita, Cherap's daughter, held an umbrella over my shoulder to shield me from others' bad thoughts.* Lhakpa, Cherap's wife, acting as my mother, showed me

---

* What I needed was an umbrella inside me, protecting me from my own bad thoughts.

where to stand and who to serve first. Whereas an American wedding felt to me like an entertainment in a Roman colosseum, with spectators watching you in the ring, this felt like the folding together of community. The entire affair was draped with loving exchanges of practicality mixed with tradition. My white dress and bouquet in Idaho felt like far more of a costume than anything I was doing here.

When it was over, I just wanted to stay in the bed at Cherap and Lhakpa's house. I wanted to have all my friends leave me there and let me get reacquainted with the distance I was used to holding between us. But I had offered this trip, and it had to go on.

Over the next ten days, Jon, our friends, and I ate Sherpa food and drank Sherpa tea and crossed the most beautiful high mountain passes in the world. I felt the slow agony of being split in half, sharing this special place even as I wanted to keep it to myself. I could hear myself being far too defensive with Jon, sniping at him when he would ask me for anything. I resisted the closeness he offered and pushed him toward my friend Amy, then watched them laugh and joke about movie quotes with ease. I hated movies. I hated this.

We got blessed by the main Lama who blesses climbers and we mingled with other guides and climbers as we approached Base Camp. I introduced my friends to Reinhold Messner when we crossed paths with him just below our destination. Jon had read about all the big names in mountaineering, and he formed opinions of them based on that prior to ever meeting one of them, which I'd learned was a quirk of his. Reinhold was a stern and stoic hero, he determined. Conrad Anker was curious and a philosophic badass. Dave Hahn was a blundering idiot. Simone Moro was feminine and loud and prototypically Italian. "That dude needs to be punched," Jon quipped about Ueli Steck, after having seen his film *The Swiss Machine*. I listened to Jon's opinions of people who I knew and he only knew of. The way he spoke of my community felt like a violation. I didn't want him to have an opinion at all. He didn't deserve one. I said nothing, though, and just let my two realities exist side by side. These people he was labeling knew me better than he ever would, and that truth stung me. It made me wonder why I had brought him there in the first place.

The day that my friends flew away was one I had been looking forward to since before we even left the U.S. Aloneness would be mine again. I could focus on the season without having to explain anything to anyone or take care of anyone but myself. They departed and I sat quietly, alone, at a teahouse just below Base Camp. Tshering Dorjee, who had climbed with me in 2008 and 2010, would be my partner. Soon we would start our season of carrying loads and climbing Everest together—hopefully without oxygen for me. I drank tea all afternoon until the darkness came and sent me to my little bed in the back of the teahouse, finally feeling free.

* * *

After some time alone in the mountains, I made my way to Base Camp. My tent was at the terminus of the glacier, the very top. From the first tents of camp, it would take an hour to get to my camp, maybe more if I stopped to talk to friends. The first tent I passed was Simone's. We had become good friends after he had agreed to fly to Baruntse in the helicopter to try to help find Chhewang's body after the accident. He had been a constant companion and source of entertainment for me the previous spring, in 2012, when I was working with Dave Hahn and he was attempting to climb the West Ridge with a separate team. Part of the levity he brought came from his Italian-to-English translations, which were never perfect but always funny. Near the end of our season in 2012, I texted him asking if he would bring our team a box of wine on his next heli. The boxed wine was cheap, horrible Nepali wine, but it lasted the season and was easy to transport. Simone agreed, but when he arrived at our camp the next day, he marched in with a cardboard box carrying eight glass bottles of wine. "I am a fucking Italian! I cannot see you drink wine out of a box! The only thing worse is French wine!"

That was Simone. He had a larger-than-life ego and sense of himself in space. Simone wasn't the center of the world; he *was* the world. We all lived and breathed because of him so generously allowing us to do so. I found this endlessly entertaining more than annoying, watching him get worked up at the smallest things and misinterpreting nearly everything else. We had a mother-child relationship dynamic, and he enjoyed being taken care of by me as much as I enjoyed being the voice of reason for him.

I entered the camp for some tea and to meet his climbing partners. He was planning to climb the West Ridge, but even more ambitiously, he would then descend the Southeast Ridge and climb Lhotse to complete a horseshoe climb, one that had never been done before. The climb was the idea and dream of the great Ueli Steck, who had brought a team that consisted of Simone and a filmmaker and friend, Jonathan Griffith. I had only met Ueli briefly in 2010, but I had seen him moving quickly in the mountains, verifying to me that the hype was true. He was an animal, but a mysterious one to me.

In addition to their team of three, they were sharing a base camp with Simone's longtime climbing partner and friend, Denis Urubiko. Denis was Russian born, and a true hardman, climbing 8,000-meter peaks by new routes, without oxygen, mostly in winter. Since Simone was committed to climb with Ueli, Denis's partner for this season was a fellow Russian hardman,* Alexey Bolotov. A schoolteacher off the mountain, Alexey saved his money for years at a time to fund these improbable adventures with Denis. Both of them were behemoths, with fingers thicker than beer brats, and deep weathered lines in their faces. They didn't speak much English, but it didn't matter, because they didn't speak much at all. They weren't here to chat; they were here to climb. I had tea and introduced myself to this tent of badasses, with Simone doing most of the talking.

It would be more than a week before I saw them again. They were

---

* Is that redundant? If you are Russian, are you automatically a hardman? I have never met a soft Russian, but I am sure they exist.

ahead of me on their acclimatization, and I had heard rumors from the Sherpas that they were climbing through the icefall with only tennis shoes and trekking poles, practically running. I imagined they would have to run to avoid all the amateur climbers who wanted a photo with them, especially Ueli, who had become famous outside the niche climbing world after the *Swiss Machine* film chronicled his speed records on the Eiger in Switzerland. Like most people at the camps, I was curious about him. In my brief interactions he had seemed stern, and shy. But I wanted to break through that and ask him questions about his climb without oxygen the previous year. I wanted to get his take on the late-season weather patterns. I mostly just wanted him to acknowledge me as a real climber, since that was what I aspired to be.

After a few weeks of climbing and resting at camp, I texted Simone to see if I could join them for dinner, as I knew they were down from one of their glacier runs. He welcomed me with the fantastic, over-excited expressions of both an Italian and a lonely man at a base camp with few women. I was the public service Simone could provide his team—a real-life girl! Through the dinner Simone dominated the conversation, interrupted occasionally by Jonathan's quick wit. It was a nice break from all my solo time, as much as I was enjoying being alone. "Tomorrow we will take Simone's heli down to Namche," Ueli said in a calm and quiet voice. "You should come. The weather is shit for some days." I wanted to, badly, but I was supposed to be waiting for a writer from *Men's Journal* who was trekking in and wanted to interview me. Simone told me to think about it and decide tomorrow, but in any case I should come back and have breakfast with them. As he walked me out, he said, "See, Meli, I think you prove to him you are okay!" *Prove what to whom?* I wondered. But he went on, as Simone always did. "He thinks you are . . . How do you say?" He paused, bringing his index finger to his nose and pushing it into the air. "An elitist! But I tell him you are not. You are Meli. You are wonderful and now tonight I think he see my way. He invite you to come down with us, so I think he see my way."

Simone proclaimed victory as I slowly began to understand what he was saying. Ueli thought I was an elitist! He thought I was stuck up? I flashed on my husband Jon saying that someone needed to punch that guy. How was *I* stuck up? *He* was the one with the elitist ego. I felt the little rage rise in me. I didn't have to prove myself to anyone. I decided then that I wouldn't go with them to Namche. I didn't need elitist Ueli Steck judging me.

When morning came, I made my way to their camp to tell them to fly without me. Simone was in the shower tent and the Russians were somewhere, but never in the shower.* Jonathan was still sleeping in his tent, and so that left only Ueli and me. Ueli was quiet and precise in his every movement. I sensed that the stoic exterior wasn't all there was to him, but it was hard to know. His hands were callused with the knotty knuckles of a rock climber, but he didn't wear the typical climber attire. His clothes were clean and free from the normal duct-tape patches that many of the other climbers' jackets had. His face was clean-shaven and his hair was washed, not greasy from a long, showerless expedition. He wasn't a dirtbag—he was a professional, taking all of this very seriously.

Standing there with him and thinking of what he'd said of me, I immediately felt awkward, angry. "You take some strong coffee?" he said quietly, pointing to the Italian coffee machine Simone had assembled.

"Sure." I was torn about what to do: Should I not talk? Should I start talking a lot? I wanted him to know that I wasn't stuck up at all. I wanted him to know that I was just intimidated by him.

His words interrupted my thoughts. "So, you come with us, okay? If you want to climb without oxygen, you need rest and food. The weather will be shit for three days, so come with us. We can do some nice running."

"I want to . . ." I said tentatively, "but—there is this journalist coming any day, and I should wait for him."

Ueli shook his head. "No, you don't let them control you, or they

---

* Part of being a Russian hardman is that you cannot do anything that brings comfort during an expedition or you will get soft.

will. You tell him you go down. He wants to talk to you, he comes down too. Don't let them tell you what to do."

It was settled. It felt good to be told what to do by him, like the mentorship I had craved but never found. I would join them. I ran back up to my camp to pack for a few nights away. I let Tshering know my plan, promising to bring some fresh chicken and greens back to camp when I returned.

The day was spent in Ueli and Simone's base camp, perfectly perched next to the helipad. We laughed and lounged and drank coffee while waiting for the helicopter to take us to Namche. I was sure it wasn't going to come as I watched the evening clouds roll in and overtake everything. But just as the sun was almost gone, the giant booming rotors descended from an impossibly small hole in the clouds and swooped us up. In the helicopter it took only a few moments to deliver us to thick air and ground that would have taken three days to cover on foot. We stumbled out of the helicopter; Ueli, Simone, and me—somewhere between Ueli's tag-along little sister and Simone's mother. Ueli handed me my backpack, commenting on how Americans always carried such heavy backpacks. "But maybe it is because they also have nice picnics in the mountains." I couldn't tell if it was an insult or a compliment, but I felt self-conscious either way.

As we sat down for a pasta dinner in Namche, Simone slinked to the kitchen of the teahouse to find some red wine for us. I picked up my fork and spoon and twirled the pasta in the way I always had. Ueli smiled. "You better not let Simone see you eat pasta with a spoon—he won't let you on the heli again. He is very Italian, you know."

I responded without thinking. "I am not stuck up!" He was taken aback. I could see it. "Simone told me you said I was elitist."

He nodded and looked me straight in the eye. "I understand who you are. You have to be that way, or how could you survive as a girl with all these guys? It is the only way. I understand."

He put to words the purpose of my hard exterior. He recognized my need to survive. I was starting to see the human under the superhero

climber. Ueli was funny in a sly little way that required you to pay attention. He was thoughtful, too, with more layers than I initially suspected.
And he was obviously driven and focused. But contrary to what Jon
said, he didn't need to be punched at all. In that moment of sharing
pasta etiquette and my fear of being seen, he held up a mirror to show
me that my reflection was the outline of his. We were more similar than
we were different.

Over the next days, the three of us laughed, ate as much food as we
could, and ran through the trails surrounding the 12,000-foot village.
When I was there a few weeks before for my Sherpa wedding, I'd felt
confined and tethered. But now I felt free, like I was growing into the
person I wanted to be. I was understood. No one needed an explanation
for my drive to be here in these big mountains. Ueli told me how he
used shakes and powders for recovery when up high. He showed me the
mask he used to cover his face and keep his throat from getting too dry
while climbing without oxygen. We laughed with (and at) Simone, so-
lidifying our trio and the newly formed bonds of friendship. I felt more
than included. I felt like I belonged.

* * *

After we returned to Everest Base Camp, the season continued as
planned, as I prepared to make my summit bid without oxygen. I made
my way up to Camp One with Tshering and eventually onward to Camp
Two. We carried tents and oxygen for Tshering and cans of fuel. Tshering, being Sherpa, didn't need to acclimatize as much as I did, so I made
various journeys up the mountain to Camp Two alone while he stayed
at Base Camp playing cards.

On the night of April 26, I was alone at Camp Two once again,
preparing to head to Camp Three in the coming days, once the route
had fixed lines in place and Tshering had rejoined me. The weather had
been finicky, and so the team of Sherpas who fixed the rope had been
slowed, mostly waiting while hanging around Camp Two. Ueli and

Jonathan and Simone were also in Camp Two that night, planning to climb to Camp Three the next day (without the fixed lines) and sleep one night up high. I joined them for dinner. Ueli cooked a Swiss rosti and I made it an American rosti by adding bacon, to Ueli's approval. As we drank tea after dinner and lounged in the big dome tent they were using, Jonathan told us dirty jokes and we laughed until it hurt. I couldn't take any more laughter, so I bid them goodnight, heading to my own little tent to sleep while they dogpiled together in the big dome.

Early the next morning I migrated back uphill for breakfast with them. They were eager to get going and I rushed them out of the tent, assuring them I would clean it up so they could get climbing before it got too warm. I did the dishes and packed away the food, feeling included rather than demeaned by being allowed to clean up camp. I felt like they saw me as important to their team, even though I wasn't *on* their team. Tshering was my partner, and we had climbed together for years, but ours was a quiet partnership of upward movement. With Ueli and Simone, I felt camaraderie. I was learning how to climb like them and mimic their graceful mountain movements.

As they climbed up the face, closer and closer to the large team of Sherpas who were fixing ropes, I headed downhill to my friend Phunuru Sherpa's camp for coffee, plunking myself in a wobbly chair on the ice next to him. We sat sipping coffee and watching the climbers on the steep Lhotse face, when suddenly an American guide called over the radio to say that some climbers were stupidly trying to climb on the fixed ropes while the Sherpas were placing them, but he had successfully told them to turn around. The guide also said that Ueli and Simone* were way out in the middle of the face, moving fast and not a problem for the Sherpas who were working. The radios quieted and we sat with our coffee in the hot sun of Camp Two.

---

* No one ever included Jonathan in their descriptions, even though he was always there. He was very much the forgotten climber of that team.

Suddenly the radio sparked to life with Nepali chatter. When Nepalis call you on the radio, they scream as though the tent is on fire no matter what they are saying, almost as though they mistrust the radio's power. But the yelling today sounded uniquely angry. I watched Phunuru squinting up at the slope as he yelled back at the radio. "What is it?" I asked, hoping there hadn't been an accident.

"The Sherpas are done. They are coming down. They said Ueli and Simone kicked ice down and . . ." He was interrupted by more frantic radio calls. One of the American guides with us at the camp grabbed the radio and called to the other American who was on the face. "Tell those guys to come down," he commanded, though I wasn't sure if he meant Ueli and Simone or the Sherpa team.

The voice of the guide on the face crackled back: "Yeah, I don't think I can tell them anything."

A moment later, the Nepalis exploded back on the radio. In the background, I heard Simone, speaking half in Sherpa, half in Italian, punctuated by an English word here and there.

I asked for the radio so I could tell Simone to stop yelling and just come down—he would listen to me, I promised. But it was too late. Simone's voice came over the radio: "The Sherpas are very mad. I say a bad word, so they come down now." And then, silence. Silence on the radio and silence around us. Phunuru and I looked at each other, knowing that a quiet this expansive meant that it wasn't over at all.

When Simone said "I say a bad word," he wasn't saying the half of it. He and Ueli had been out in the middle of the face but they had eventually wound up higher than the Sherpas fixing the ropes, a breach of mountain protocol. And then it became clear that, in getting argumentative with the Sherpas, Simone had used a word you never, ever say in Sherpa language. And there was no taking it back.

I returned to my camp, filled with worry for how tense this situation was getting. I tried to contact Ueli and Simone on their radio. When I finally got them, Ueli told me that he and Simone had merely finished fixing the rope that the Sherpas left so that the expedition leaders wouldn't be upset. I cringed at his words. He meant well, but essentially, I was hearing him say, *I did the work the Sherpas didn't.* I told him that they should come down and talk to the Sherpa team leaders here in camp, that things were tense down here. The Nepali teams were huddling together and talking ever louder as the rope-fixing team described what had happened on the face. The sky was beginning to darken with the threat of an afternoon storm, and I had the feeling something far worse was coming. I pleaded with Simone to come down. He told me they would.

As I collapsed onto my sleeping bag, an exhale stuck in my throat. Why did Simone have to keep talking? Why did he have to say that word?*

As they arrived at camp, still climbing in their quick and graceful way, I went immediately to their tent. I tried to explain to them that it was a bigger deal than just climbing above the fixing team. Ueli said he had never been told in the mountains when he could or couldn't climb. He had had a good relationship with the Sherpas, and this seemed so bizarre to him. He just didn't understand. I could see the confusion in his bright blue eyes. Nothing was adding up to him, and it spread an air of confusion to us all. Just then, one of the American leaders, Greg, entered the tent. His words were firm and accusing. "You guys messed up. You can't climb when the boys are working. You messed up." He was over six feet tall and towered over both Simone and Ueli, neither of them taller than five-nine.

Ueli defended himself in a much quieter tone. "Yeah, I don't understand this. I climb everywhere and no one says you can't climb. We didn't touch the ropes!"

As they exchanged words without understanding, I slipped out of the tent. A moment later I heard a rumbling, the commotion of a stam-

---

* The word Simone used directly translates to "motherfucker," but in Sherpa it is never a casual word or a joke. Even when the Sherpas teach Westerners bad words, they tell them *never* to say that one, and Simone knew this.

pede. Looking up, I saw over a hundred Sherpas* moving en masse up the hill toward Ueli and Simone's camp. Their jackets were a brightly colored collage of movement and their heads were covered with warm winter hats, bobbing up the glacier in the wave of a rising tide. I turned around and rushed back into the tent. "Can you control your staff?" I asked Greg, urgently. He shook his head as his eyes narrowed. No, he couldn't. I believed him. The group of Sherpas had gotten too large, too angry. No one could talk to them now.

I looked at Ueli, whose bright eyes were wide and wet with concern. "I don't want to be dramatic, but you guys need to get the fuck out of here. Run up the glacier, just go. There is a huge group coming up and they are angry, and I don't know what will happen!" I was out of breath, feeling the flood of anxiety exit my chest through my words.

Jonathan and Ueli and Simone fled the tent just as the mass arrived. Loud words turned to chaotic yelling and the commotion of so many people overtook the normally calm space of Camp Two. Time moved so fast, and events unfolded so unpredictably, that it felt like the only thing anyone could do was react. Groups of Sherpas huddled together, incensed, their voices raised. I begged them, hands clasped together in prayer, for no violence. Suddenly my eyes alit on a rock the size of a dinner plate arcing through the air, headed toward a blue tent. A split second later, I realized that Ueli was standing in front of that tent. I was shocked to see him standing there. He hadn't gotten away. The fastest climber on the mountain hadn't been fast enough to escape. He took another rock to the face and crumpled into a heap on the ground. The Sherpas swept in to surround him, kicking at his curled-up body. I lunged in front of him, yelling, "No violence!" and shoved him into the blue tent behind us. I didn't know whose it was, but it didn't matter. Ueli was inside, and I was outside, and I wasn't letting anyone through. I asked another guide to go to my tent and get my first-aid kit. Ueli was

---

* Mostly climbing Sherpas, but cooks and some clients who wanted to watch too.

bleeding and I wasn't sure how much worse things were going to get. I stood my ground in front of the door, my hands alternating from the Namaste prayer hands to holding tightly to Phunuru's hands. He was a Sherpa, but he was joining me in creating a barrier between the anger of the other Sherpas and Ueli. I held his hands tightly and thought about how it takes a certain type of courage to stand against the people who expect you to always stand with them.

As the yelling and rock-throwing calmed, the demands became clear: Send Simone out to apologize. I promised I would get him. He would apologize, I said, but there couldn't be any more violence. They said Simone and Ueli had to leave, go home. They said Simone had to take his helicopter home or they would destroy it. I agreed to everything they asked as Simone made his way down the glacier from the spot he was hiding. He slipped into the big dome tent and I faced him there.

"You have to go out, get on your knees, and say 'I'm sorry.'" My tone was firm; there was no room to negotiate. "Say nothing else. If they ask you something, just say 'I'm sorry.' Do you understand?" I held my hand tightly on his shoulder and looked him directly in the eye. This was serious and I wanted him to tell me he understood.

"I am not fucking getting on my knees . . ." he started to whine.

"Simone. *Yes. You. Are.* Do it." My voice rose with each word.

Finally, he nodded, and I pulled him by his arm out of the tent. The mass of Nepalis had pushed the most vocal voices forward. I used their names and begged them again not to be violent. As Simone stepped forward out of the tent, I growled at him in a quiet tone with conviction, "Get on your knees." He resisted until one of the Sherpas came close, screaming in his face that he had to leave and take his helicopter. They didn't like him, and he wasn't welcome. This wasn't the beginning of their issues with Simone. He was loud and boisterous, which was generally discouraged in the quiet communities of Sherpas working in the mountains. He had also made promises about not charging Nepalis for helicopter flights and then reneged when it came time to fly them. So their disdain wasn't a complete surprise, but the intensity of the eruption was. I pushed his shoulder down, and as soon as he kneeled, the front row of Sherpas began to kick at him. As he started to say a quiet "I am sorry," one of them stepped forward and slapped him across the face.

The promise of no more violence had been clearly broken. I yelled at everyone as I put myself in front of Simone, pushing him back into the tent. My voice was firm. "That's it. They will leave, but you have to leave too. It is over!" I recognized the small power I had in that moment and knew my words would be heeded, though I wasn't sure why. Phunuru added Sherpa words to reinforce mine and slowly the assembled Sherpas started making their way downhill and away from the conflict. It ended just as surprisingly as it had begun.

I went back into the blue tent to check on Ueli. He was okay physically, just bleeding from a cut in his mouth. But in his eyes, I could tell he was changed; he was shaken. There was a gray veil over the normally crystal-blue bulbs. I looked at him, holding his gaze but unsure what I could say.

He, Simone, and Jonathan quickly packed their bags and collapsed their tent. They headed out to the center of the glacier, a dangerous but hidden descent route. As they fled Camp Two that season, I made my way through camp to talk with the Sherpas and tell them I was sorry for how the situation had escalated. The thin air felt heavy, and very few words were exchanged. My mind was abuzz with what I had just seen. Never could I have imagined things would go this way. I felt like it wasn't real, a bad dream, and the fog of altitude combined with so much surprise was amplifying that feeling.

After a restless night at Camp Two, I decided to descend. I arrived at Base Camp to over a hundred messages in my email, phone, and satellite phone from people I knew and journalists I didn't, all wanting to know what happened. Headlines read, "American Girl Saves Climbers from Angry Mob of Sherpas." For a moment I wondered how the news had gotten out, but then I knew it was Simone. He would be the teller of this tale. And he had a lot to say.

The elder Sherpas around camp were appalled and embarrassed.

They wanted things back to normal fast, and to this end, they helped to write a peace agreement with Ueli, Simone, and Jonathan. Everyone would admit responsibility. Everyone would apologize and drape white blessing scarves on each other's necks, shake hands, and take pictures. Those pictures were to be sent to the press so people could forget that this very bad day ever happened. There would be peace.

But no one would forget. Ueli went home, quietly and quickly, only to be vilified by the Swiss press. Jonathan left just as quickly, resigned to believe that Everest was the circus everyone said it was. Simone, though, stayed and kept flying his helicopter, forcing his presence whether it was wanted or not. His base camp would stay up, still hosting Denis and Alexey. The leaders of the Sherpa staff would struggle with threats from the rest of the staff that if any of the more aggressive Sherpas were fired they would all quit.

I tucked myself back in at my own camp, now quiet and lonely without my adoptive European team. For the remainder of April and beginning of May, I stayed at Base Camp, harassed by emails from the media and tortured by my own questioning if I wanted to even stay.[*] But ultimately, I decided that the only way through it was to continue. I had felt this way after Chhewang died and I was considering quitting climbing altogether. If I stopped when things were so bad, I would never be able to change them. They would stay bad forever. So up I would go, slowly trying to regain the magic I had felt when I was part of that team. Because I had wanted so badly to be alone that season, it came as a surprise to me that I was mourning the loss of a team. The difference between what you want and what you need always seems to

---

[*] The sketchy media had gotten my husband Jon's phone number and called him, telling him that I had said it was okay for him to relay my version of the events to them. I, meanwhile, continued to decline to talk. Who was I to summarize something so complicated? Who was I to give information to allow people to decide who was good and who was bad? Who was an elitist and who was a savage? I couldn't do it then and I still struggle to do it now. I have a hard time telling the story with anything other than the simplest facts, as you have just read.

emerge when you are busy doing something else. It was emerging for me now.

The season continued. Acclimatization continued. The jet stream came and then receded, and the summit bids began. Tshering and I were ready. I had stayed in touch with Ueli via messages on the sat phone. He gave me weather forecasts and told me to go for it. He had fully become the mentor I had so deeply wanted Ed Viesturs to be four years earlier. Early in the trip Ueli had taken me running with him, showing me how he kept his fitness up while waiting to climb. He shared information before I had to ask, so I never felt like I was annoying him with my curiosity. He gave me firm but gentle encouragement. As a young woman in climbing, I had been so afraid to ask for help, for fear of seeming weak, and Ueli saw that and offered what he could before I could ask. But my heart was broken that he couldn't be here too. I had wanted to climb near him and learn even more about how he managed to be so resilient at very high altitude.

When the time for our summit bid arrived in late May, three weeks after the fight, Tshering and I spent a long day climbing from Camp Two all the way to Camp Four to take advantage of what was supposed to be a good-weather window. But when we arrived at the South Col, the wind was unrelenting and a fine mist of snow coated everything. We tucked into the tent, vowing to venture back out in the middle of the night when the wind often calmed. But as ten p.m. turned to midnight, the winds continued. We decided to go out anyway, knowing that we were the only climbers attempting it that night and knowing that the wind often died once a climber reached the base of the face. To get to the face we had to traverse a blank and open glacier to find the start of the fixed lines. The wind was violent, throwing us to our knees every few steps, but we continued forward, hopeful. As the slope began to steepen, I yelled to Tshering, asking if he could see the fixed lines. He could not. And I could not. We were at the spot where part of the 1996 team had died, in the thin air, so close to camp but unable to get there. "I think we should go down," I said, heavy with the knowledge that this

was likely our only chance at the summit.* Tshering agreed, and we retreated to the noisy flapping fabric of our tent, caught in a windstorm.
Tshering quickly fell asleep as I lay there awake, with Alexey Bolotov's
name caught in the hamster wheel of my mind.

Alexey Bolotov. Alexey Bolotov. Alexey Bolotov.

At first light I started the stove and told Tshering I thought we
should go down and rest. Maybe we would be able to come back up. I
also told him I had Alexey's name stuck in my head. I asked him if that
ever happened to him, getting one word or phrase stuck in his head.

"Like a prayer, you mean?" His question reminded me that much of
being a monk was chanting the same words again and again.

Tshering was quieter than usual as we drank tea and headed down.
We were moving slowly, descending as most other climbers came up,
each asking if we made it. After hours of this, I asked him if he was
okay. He said he never tried to go to the summit only to turn around,
and he was sad. I promised we would try again. We still had time. We
could rest and then we would try again. I was surprised that he cared
about the summit at all, but it made me feel good to know that he did.
We had that in common, a little thread to remind us that we were both
here for something.

As we stumbled, tired and wind-burnt, into Camp Two, I pulled the
sat phone out of my pack and powered it on. *Ding. Ding. Ding.* The
messages made their way in. Ueli, Ueli, Simone. I opened the first from
Ueli, a note that the forecast was changing and we should wait because
the winds weren't going to get low enough. True story, just a little late to
be of any help.

---

* But it wasn't. We would descend and rest and head back up, surprisingly recovered. I
would try to climb without oxygen, but we would end up using it, failing once again at
my goal, letting myself down and feeling like I let Ueli down too. Tshering and I would
summit together again, my fifth and Tshering's tenth. We would quickly descend all the
way to Camp Two the same day, and most people would consider our season a success.
But as we turned around in the pre-dawn cold and wind of that night, we didn't know
any of that, and the decision to go down felt like the finale to our difficult season.

The next two messages, one from Ueli and one from Simone, said the same thing. "Alexey died this morning." No more info.

My whole body shivered as I went and told Tshering. He told me that he had just heard that as well. Apparently, Alexey's rope had broken early that morning as he was trying to rappel at the edge of the icefall. I didn't know Alexey Bolotov, but I was certain that even though he was already dead, he had been up there at the South Col with us in the pre-dawn dark, trying to make me aware of him. How else could I explain it? I have always thought that the thin air of high altitude allows you to be closer to the spirits in the universe, and now I was surer than ever. Sometimes the heaviest things can only come through the thinnest air. And this season was full of the heaviest things.

15.

ESCAPE

2013: Rainier to Chamonix

I quickly shoved my boots into the top of my overstuffed duffel bag. They were still damp from that morning's summit, but I hoped the dryer sheets that I had stuffed inside them would help with the stench of damp boots stored in a dark bag for twelve hours. I didn't have time to do anything else—I had to go. My flight to Geneva was taking off at nine p.m. and I was still two hours from the airport, toasting my clients after a successful climb of Rainier. It had been an all-women climb. And this climb was special, my hundredth summit of the mountain. I had been guiding every summer for nine years, dutifully roping myself up with clients and gently stepping my way across the sprawling glaciers and broken, rust-colored rock. I had turned around plenty of times because of weather or to take a client down. I had summited with no food and water, with a 103-degree fever, and in a full blizzard. I had seen countless fiery pink sunrises puncture the night sky. The topography of Rainier had blended itself into my DNA and made up much of who I was.

But after one hundred climbs, I was taking a break. I had spent the last six springs on Everest, climbing and guiding and learning. Each summer, I returned dutifully to Rainier, which was both prison and liberation. It was a mountain I loved and a place that freed me, but also somewhere I felt I had to return to or else my carefully matrixed life would crumble. But this July, I decided I was going to stop making excuses and start pushing outside my comfort zone. I was going to step down from the lectern and stop being the teacher in exchange for being a student again. This was, of course, also a convenient excuse to once again run away from the life I was supposed to be building.

I had returned home to Idaho after the fight on Everest and Alexey's death with a skinny body and a heavy heart. Everyone wanted a story— what had really happened with Ueli, Simone, and the Sherpas? I couldn't tell if I even knew. I felt like a stranger, to my friends and especially to Jon. I tried to force myself back into the life I had chosen. I tried to remember all the reasons I chose marriage and this place, but my mind felt chaotic and like I had left part of myself somewhere else.

I felt further away from Jon than I ever had. He met me with what felt like the same invasive and naive curiosity that the media had. What happened in the fight? Were those Euros to blame? Was it ego? Why did it matter that I used oxygen—it was a fifth summit! I bristled at his attempts to understand me but gave him no insights to change his view. I felt more protective and wanted more distance than I ever had.

He was trying, but I was putting up walls and reinforcing every crack. He asked me if we could climb Rainier together, on a more technical route than the standard one I had guided him on previously. I agreed as I tried to hide my disdain for his lack of competency in the mountains and I helped him with the most basic tasks. I felt bad for how harshly I was judging him and his earnest attempts to connect with me in the environment I loved, but it was the only way I could justify resisting his love without admitting that I felt undeserving of it in the first place. It allowed me to hold the illusion of having the upper hand. I had been making the joke regularly when people asked if my husband was a climber, that no, I was smarter than to marry another climber. But in moments like these I wished he was. I was forgetting all the things that I had seen in him when he came into my life just three years prior. I was testing how much he would tolerate between us. I knew it was selfish. I hated being this person. But I didn't know what else to do.

And so even though I knew I should spend time with my new husband and my friends—that I should take stock and work on the healing I knew I needed; that I should continue to press myself to live with the vulnerability and address the pain that kept accreting in layers on my soul—instead of doing all that, I decided to go back to the mountains. Instead of spending our first wedding anniversary together with Jon, I booked a trip to Europe. And just as he had since before our wedding, he said nothing. But I could see in his eyes that he wished I would stay.

* * *

Since my return, Ueli and I had kept in close contact via WhatsApp messages and sat phone texts. He spoke to me like a big brother, and I felt like an annoying little sister, soliciting his advice as often as I could. He told me I needed to come to the Alps in the summer for some big climbs. He told me not to bring my giant "American backpack." The thought of going to a place I had never been and pushing myself to learn a whole new way of moving uphill (fast, not slow!) terrified me. But that was how I knew I needed to do it. In my life, I could trace all the best moments, mostly in the mountains, and see the intense discomfort that just preceded them. The thought of flying alone to France and joining a rotating list of partners on fast, challenging climbs in the Alps felt supremely uncomfortable. I couldn't wait to see what would happen next.

I boarded my red-eye and fell into the quick and deep sleep of a cat indifferent to location. When I opened my eyes, my mouth felt sticky and dry, and my neck was stiff from leaning against the window. My right side was cramped from the unnatural crunch of nine hours of flight. But immediately, I felt awake, and alive. Out the window of the plane I could see the sun rising over the French Alps and pouring its golden light into them, depositing little gifts of glitter for me to go and collect.

I landed in Geneva and exited the plane into a world that made my heart do joyful little calisthenics against my chest. This was Switzerland. I had never been, but instantly I felt like I might never leave. Everything was orderly and clean and quaint. I found a shuttle to Chamonix, France, one of the alpine adventure capitals of the world, nestled in the direct center of the French Alps and bordered closely by both Italy and Switzerland. I texted my friends Damian and Willie Benegas, Argentinian brothers, institutions in the climbing world, who would be my first European climbing partners. The Benegases had more first ascents between them than nearly anyone, and after years of spring guiding on Everest together, we had grown close. They were identical twins and hard to tell apart, though I prided myself on knowing which was which. Their personalities were so big, they always felt almost cartoonish, punctuated by the fact that they spoke a rough mix of English and Spanish. They had promised to show me how climbing in the Alps worked before turning me over to Ueli for grander adventures.

My hopes for coffee and baguettes and strolling the lovely cobbled streets of Chamonix evaporated as soon as I entered Damian and Willie's apartment. "Chica! Pack your bag!" said Damian. "If we leave now, we can get the last tram and climb tonight! We will climb the Gervasutti!"

I panicked, trying to think of a quick way out. What was the Gervasutti? My packed boots were still wet from the summit of Rainier less than twenty-four hours earlier. What if the climb was too hard for me? Sure, I had summited Everest five times, but a quick look in the guidebook told me that this was a vertical tower of rock shooting straight at the sky. This was harder. This was technical rock climbing in the alpine zone,* high above the glaciers below. What about my cheese and wine and crunchy baguette? But no excuse came quickly enough, so I agreed to go. Anyway, I hadn't come here to say no. I had come to learn and grow, which meant not making excuses to avoid the things that scared me.

What kind of climb was it? It was a twenty-five-pitch rock climb that was accessed from a glacier and would spit us out near the summit of Mount Blanc, at 15,777 feet the highest point in the Alps. From there we would descend back to the hut and ride the tram back to town again. The whole thing normally took three days, but we would try to do it in just over one. I was skeptical that I would be able to climb that many pitches of rock (roughly 2,000 feet of it), but Damian seemed to believe in me, and I believed in him, so off we went.

The climb was spectacular. It was the hardest and most incredible thing I had ever done. We started out on the sheer granite face, weaving our way up through a series of cracks and ledges. Willie would lead the rope and Damian and I would climb as quickly as we could behind him. The sun came up and warmed our fingers, spreading its warm orange light on the tan and black rocks. We climbed pitch after pitch, snaking our way up, up, up over a thousand vertical feet. Birds soared around us in the sky as we moved in unison. The difficult rock climbing brought us up a beautiful spire that exited onto a perfect glacier ridge. The slope dropped down thousands of feet on one side and gently rolled away on the other and we traversed our way across the snow-and-ice ridge dividing the two. We roped up to scurry as quickly as we could over the crevasses and ice ledges of the glacier back to the hut. We had spent the day laughing together at the anchors and climbing quickly as a team of three. I pulled myself over each ledge and delicately stepped across each face with the glacier a thousand feet below me. My feet were sore from being shoved inside rock shoes all day, but my heart swelled with such happi-

---

* The alpine is defined by the area above the tree line, marked by rock, ice, and thinner air.

ness that I couldn't feel anything else. I was doing it! This was the magic of climbing—when it was hard, the pain could make you forget any other pain in your life, and when it was good, the blossoms of joy would crowd out any other emotions.

When we descended back to Chamonix, I texted Ueli to let him know I was there. He told me he would arrive the next day and we could have dinner and go for a climb. I felt curious to see how he was doing since the fight. It was impossible to tell from our text exchanges, but I was hoping he was okay. I told him where I was staying, a sweet little French hostel now that the Benegas brothers had left the country.

Ueli met me in the lobby. I walked down to find him surrounded by a small group asking for photos and autographs. As I approached, he broke away from them, giving me a warm hug and a grateful look. But something was still wrong with his eyes.

Everything about Ueli seemed larger than life and impenetrable, leading the media to call him the Swiss Machine. He wasn't very tall, only five-eight, but he seemed to tower over everyone. His legs were un-naturally bowed, a remnant of a hip defect when he was born. But those legs danced effortlessly up hills and over rocks and stuck to sheer ice with the grace of a dancer. He had hands that were twice as big as mine, making everything feel small next to them. His jaw was sharp and firm, suggesting further impenetrability. But his eyes always betrayed the machine-like exterior. They were the crystal blue of a melted glacier pool, looking both mesmerizing and unreal. Framed by dark eyebrows full of emotion, they were often wet. If you saw Ueli climb, you might believe he was a machine. But if you saw his eyes, you would know that he was no machine at all. And now, looking at his eyes in the well-lit lobby of my Chamonix hostel, I could see he wasn't okay.

There is something that happens with friendships formed in the thin air of high altitude—they operate on an accelerated timeline. Life in the mountains is distilled down to the simplicity of movement and sur-vival. Without the distractions and comforts of daily life, you end up showing your whole self to the mountain, both good and bad, and the people that surround you will get that view too, making the bond stronger than the stones you climb over. I felt that even deeper with Ueli after the fight. In those few moments in the tent, I had seen his most tender center. I had seen someone who was truly afraid and not hiding it, and in this revelation, I had seen a part of myself. We had become siblings, bonded by a moment that neither of us had wanted. I had been there on his worst day. I had stood between him and a quickly spiraling nightmare. I had watched as he left the mountain, head down in confusion.

But that was months ago, and I had hoped some time away from it would pull him back to the center and the stability he had seemed to have when I first met him. "How are you?" I asked, holding his gaze steadily and firmly, fearful that if I blinked, I might lose him.

"This is crazy. The media here is saying I am so horrible. They just keep talking and saying I am a big problem. I don't go into the mountains at all since I come home. It is just crazy." I could hear that he was tired in the way his voice whispered and broke, far different from the confident statements I was used to hearing from him. I wondered what I would do if I were him, facing all this. He was the one who had told me not to let the media control me, and it hurt to see him feeling so controlled. I wondered if I could endure even one part of what he was going through. He broke my curiosity with his own. "How are you? How is your husband?" My breath caught in my chest at his words. I was here to climb and learn, but I was also here to escape the gnawing feeling that I shouldn't have married Jon, that by doing so I had just checked another box on someone else's list.

Ueli had chosen to live his life in the mountains, in nature, following her rules. After the fight, he told me he always believed it would be the mountains that killed him, certainly not another person hurtling rocks at him from behind a nylon tent wall. The simplicity and freedom he felt in the mountains had become complex and imprisoning in one quick moment. Now that moment wouldn't leave him alone.

When he told me he was hurting, I could tell he was unafraid that I would judge him as weak. And I didn't judge him. I admired him. I had never been close to someone who was so open and vulnerable, unafraid to show the good and bad so quickly. I was used to the highly curated existence that people like Peter had shown me. Don't reveal too much. Don't be weak. Control what people see, and you will get where you want to go.

But the past three years of practicing hadn't moved me any closer to the person I wanted to be. When I looked into my own eyes, I saw the same signs of brokenness that I now saw in Ueli. I wasn't any more whole than he was. But unlike Ueli, I was afraid to admit that to anyone, even myself. Be put together. Be strong. Be impenetrable and you will be valued. Only now, seeing Ueli, did I start to consider that maybe my calculus was flawed.

My breath finally escaped my chest and I told him things were great. The previous spring on Everest he had joked that we could hang out because we were both married, so no one would question anything. It felt like the partnership I formed with Dave Morton on Everest in the early days—brother and sister. But with Ueli, I feared that he wouldn't be my friend and mentor if I let him know that my marriage was in trouble, though I wanted to share it. I wanted to open up to him in return for all he had shared with me, but instead I quickly changed the subject to the climb I had just completed.

We went to dinner and caught up about our plans for the future. "I will go to Annapurna South." He said the words, but the excitement was missing from his voice. Annapurna was situated only fifty-five miles to the east in Nepal and considered one of the deadliest 8,000-meter peaks, with a route that was far more technical than Everest. "I don't know if I should go back to Nepal or not since the fight." He shrugged and took a small bite of his salmon.

I tried to reassure him. "I think it is okay, really." The people in Nepal mostly had forgiven the incident and understood it to be as complicated as it was.

"I don't know. This climb, this is really the climb. It is so big. It would be huge. But it is very dangerous and I tell my wife I won't do solo climbs anymore, so I will go with a partner. But honestly, I don't know." He paused, and I waited, sensing what he was trying to say. "Maybe this is my last climb." He was hinting that the climb on Annapurna was so dangerous that he might not make it home. He was hinting that he was okay with that. It was a sentiment that was familiar in my own mind, but I chased it away like the ghost that it was.

When I said goodnight to Ueli and returned to my room that night, I shut the door and slid down it into a crumpled ball on the floor. It was like I had been holding my breath and holding back all night. Tears poured down my face, blurring my vision and turning the room into a surreal painting. I was crying because Ueli was broken. I was crying because I was broken, too. We had different lives and experiences, but here we were, connected by the same emotion. I cried because he could share it with me, seemingly fearless of my judgment. As I sat on the floor in Chamonix in tears, I felt weak for hiding them. I felt like a fraud. Ueli had shown his imperfection openly, and in doing that, somehow became more perfect. The hurt in his eyes, unhidden, had leapt into my core and planted a little seed. Maybe being honest and feeling things didn't make you weak. Maybe it was the lie and the shield that made you weak.

I was almost thirty years old, and this was the very first time this thought had crossed my mind. What if all the stories I told to build a fortress around my true self were just a container that was preventing me from growing into all I could be? What if I couldn't just force my way forward? What if I needed to flow instead? A dam on a river creates a deep lake in one place, but when the river flows free it changes an entire landscape. Ueli lived his life as a river flowing wherever it went. I lived mine as a dam. I wondered if I could flow like a river, changing the whole landscape. I fell asleep trying to forget the truth he was showing me but knowing I never would.

My dreams danced with my memories, as they had so many nights before. I scrolled through various scenes of the life I had lived until finally my mind stopped and I could see myself at my parents' house, a teenager the summer before I left home for good. I saw myself sitting completely still on the hard plastic porch swing, and suddenly, I was back there, in Montana on a warm summer night.

The swing was an old chairlift that my dad had scavenged from a ski resort in Colorado in the eighties, before I was born, back when he was a Kerouac-esque wanderer living with his dog in a little log cabin and soaking himself in the stillness of nature's breath. As I rocked gently in the swing, I wondered what he would be like if I had never been born. I wondered if he would be happy. By the time the hot tears hit my hands, they were cold. That seemed about right. What was in me was cold and looking for escape.

I didn't know what it felt like to be any other teenage girl, though everything I heard referenced that it was hard. Changing into a woman was hard. Navigating the social landscape of high school was hard. The new and unreasonably large feelings were hard. And I felt all of that, but I felt something else, too. I had spent the years in between childhood and becoming a woman in a rapid and unyielding descent into darkness. My mother made my non-belonging known in nearly every interaction. She created a fortress of silence between us, and I built tunnels of distance to surround her. My sixteen-year-old face had turned gaunt and pale over the preceding months and my eyes turned dark and empty. I knew I had to escape; I just didn't know what kind of escape it would be.

Earlier that day the mother bear had snarled and growled and told me to go lock myself in my room so she didn't kill me. She called me a liar. She called me a whore. I heard her voice alongside echoes of the girls in my high school taunting me in a childish way. Memories collided into one another as I heard my sister slam her door in my face and scream, "I HATE YOU!" I heard the boys I had dated tell me they didn't want to be with me after all. All the words and memories flooded my mind, turning a chaotic collision of voices into a deafening downpour of emotion. It was the sound of being unwanted. Unloved. Unlovable.

I climbed the stairs and turned into my bedroom at the top, shutting my door with a gentle click. I slid down the back of the door and hugged my knees toward my chest and let the heaviness of my head rest in my folded arms. I felt paralyzed. I felt empty. After a prolonged stillness, I pulled out my notebook and began to write. I wrote one letter to my dad and another one to everyone else. I told my dad I was sorry that I had ruined his life, and I hoped he could be happy now that I was gone. I told everyone else I didn't care if they were happy that I was gone or not—being gone meant that I was happy. I wasn't sure if these letters were runaway letters or suicide notes, but I knew that they were the first step of my escape.

I sat unmoving for hours. When the horizon absorbed the sun and the sky finally turned as dark as I felt, I went down to the porch swing. There was something nice about sitting in a darkness that felt darker than what was inside me. I thought about getting in my truck and driving. But I knew from experience that the darkness would just follow me. Darkness doesn't care about geography. I wished there were an easy and obvious way to end things. A boy a few years older than me had shot himself in his parents' garage the year before. I wished I had a gun and the knowledge to use it. As I thought about making this escape my final one, the tears that had been my constant companion ceased. I felt empty. I had nothing left to pour out. I couldn't imagine life ever feeling different from this, and I just wanted to start over. I didn't know what would happen, but I was certain that the unknown couldn't be worse than what I knew.

It was July and the crickets were chirping melodically in the grass. The air was cooling down as the night draped into every nook around me. I got up and walked to the shed behind our house. There was no door, just an old frame that opened into an even deeper darkness. There were rafters high above my head and a dirt floor under my bare feet. No one used this space; it was almost forgotten. There was a pile of extension cords attached to a work light, and a five-gallon bucket with some tools in it. I looked at the rafter and the bucket. If I flipped the bucket and used it to stand on, I could sling the cords over the rafter. I didn't know how to tie a slipknot, so I twisted and tangled the orange cord around itself until there was a loop that I could reach from on top of the bucket. I wanted to get everything just right. I would set up my exit now and then choose the perfect time to leave. I stood on the dirt floor and wondered if the cord would hold my body, suspended by only my head. I wondered if I would be able to get my head through the hole in the cord. I climbed on top of the bucket and pulled the face-size loop toward me, carefully slipping it over my head. I closed my eyes and imagined what it would feel like to leap and let my body be heavier than my head for once. My fingers wrapped around the orange cord as it slipped loosely around my neck and I stood on one foot, feeling if it would be possible to tip the bucket.

My balance shifted and the bucket slipped out from under my toes, dropping onto its cylindrical side and rolling away from me. The cord cinched on my curled fingers and around my neck, yanking the wind from my throat. This wasn't supposed to be it. This was supposed to be practice. I skittered my feet in space, begging the bucket to come closer. My right foot found it, rolled it closer to me, and allowed just enough relief to fight the imperfect noose off my neck. I collapsed onto the dirty ground and gasped, still holding my hands tightly to my neck. My fingers felt frigid and bony, and my neck felt soft and warm and alive against the cold of my hands. And then the tears came back. Relentless this time. A sudden storm with a downpour flooding my face and lap and the ground with endless soaking wetness. In that short second of uncertainty, I knew that death wasn't an escape at all. The escape was in the possibility of things being different.

I went back into the house, suddenly feeling small and like the shell of an egg that has broken open. I looked in the mirror and saw the red and purple abrasion line across my throat. I looked into my eyes, and for the first time in a long time, they didn't look so empty. The darkness had shifted. Instead of the infinite black hole that was swallowing me, it felt like an embrace.

That night I fell into a dreamless rest. When I woke up, my pain was still there. The suffocating feeling in my mother's home hadn't left. The looks of disappointment on my father's face remained. My sister still said she hated me. But the darkness was different. I had danced at the door of escape and felt the finality of it. I folded up the letters I had written and tucked them into my journal. They would be my runaway notes if they would be anything. I wondered what would happen next, and I nestled myself into that curiosity. If I died, so would curiosity. If I died, I would never know what happened next. And not knowing felt like a death of its own.

I had hoped to never see that endless darkness again. But now, fifteen years later, I had seen it in Ueli's eyes when he had hinted this might be his last climb. I had decided never to let anyone know how broken I had been. I had placed a mountain between me and the world, hoping no one would see what was truly inside but instead be distracted by the ice, snow, and glittering summit. But the mountain was starting to move and crumble, threatening to reveal me to everyone, including myself.

16.

UNAVOIDABLE

2014: Everest, Nepal

U eli went to Annapurna that fall, climbing the dangerous South Face solo in just over twenty-seven hours. But he came home, and with his return, I could exhale instead of waiting for horrible news of his death. I saw him again in the winter and his eyes had regained a small sparkle of light. He was healing. I asked him what had changed. "I just love," he said.

It was a simple concept but one that was evading me. I wished I could just love instead of feeling like I had so much to prove before that was even possible. If I could prove all the things to all the people, and myself, then I could just love. Ueli said it so simply. He made me wish that I could exist inside of that very simplicity.

The spring of 2014 I departed for my sixth expedition to Everest. I left Jon and my friends at home this time, coveting my separation more openly. The night before I left, we had drinks with Jon's friends. They remained mostly strangers to me, as I kept leaving for the mountains instead of investing in the life we had promised to build together. "Are we hosting family dinner this week?" a blond woman named Caren asked Jon from across the table. My eyes narrowed.

"Yes, let's do pancakes again," said Jon, offering her a smile. "Since neither of us can cook." Once he felt the heat of my gaze, he turned to me. "Caren has been my family dinner partner when you're gone." I nodded silently. Family dinner was something he did with his friends, the group of them rotating to a different house each week and gathering for a big joyful meal. It was what families did. But I still didn't know what it meant to be part of a family.

A day later I was a world away, in Nepal, meeting my partner, Pasang Lamu Sherpa Akita. She was a friend and one of the few female Sherpas to work in the mountains. She was born into climbing in the small village of Lukla, at the start of the trek to Everest Base Camp. After her parents' deaths while she was a teen, she took over raising her sister while finishing school and starting to work as a trekking guide. She completed courses in climbing and joined an Everest expedition in 2007, making it to the summit. We had met a few years prior and started planning an expedition together. I loved her strong and sensible calm. I loved having another woman by my side, and one who knew how it felt to take care of herself.

Now we were just two women climbing Everest together. It was our goal to do it from the Nepal side first, me without oxygen, and then descend and travel to Tibet and climb again from the north side. This double summit in one season had been done before, but never by a female team and never without oxygen. Pasang had only climbed from the north and I had only climbed from the south, so we figured we could bring our knowledge together. We were eager to challenge ourselves and make our mark.

But nearly as soon as we arrived at our camp in mid-April, things slowly started to unravel. Our climbing gear—packed in duffels and lashed to the back of a yak in a village thirty miles from Base Camp— had taken an unplanned detour and would not arrive as expected. This would delay our acclimatization and decrease our chances of getting two summits in. There was nothing we could do, so we wandered around camp, chatting with friends and drinking too much tea. We attended multiple puja ceremonies—the blessing from a Buddhist Lama before the climb. The ceremony comprised a powerful ritual. All of the climbers and workers on each team would gather around a small stone altar and sit on mattresses dragged out from the tents and spread out on the rocks and ice. Then the monks would begin their melodic chanting, reading the Tibetan scripts and asking the mountain for safe passage. Juniper burned in the center of the altar, creating a dense white smoke that floated around everything. About halfway through the blessing, various Sherpas—especially those who had previously been monks, would raise a large pole atop the altar, with long strings of prayer flags spreading outward in a star pattern from the pole to the edges of camp. The dancing would start. Beer and locally made rice beer called chang was passed around, along with platters of fruit and fried snacks. Song after song would echo through the expansive amphitheater of Base Camp as the whole team formed a swaying circle, linking arms over shoulders, feet kicking forward in a special ceremonial line dance.

Each team had their own ceremony, and we hopped from one to the next, receiving a red string from the Lama of the camp, which we tied around our necks as a blessing. Pasang and I were called the Lady Climbers by all the Nepalis, and we giggled at this name. All the local workers were planning to head up the next day to establish Camp One. The foreign guides and clients would ascend in the days that followed. Pasang and I would have been climbing the next day, too, as we had no staff, but our gear was down the trail on a lazy yak. So instead, we socialized and waited.

As we returned to our own camp that afternoon, our expedition manager, Dawa, sought me out. He looked upset. "I have terrible news," he said.

My stomach dropped at the thought of tragedy. But he had just gotten word that our visa into Tibet had been denied; something about

Obama and the Dalai Lama and Americans wouldn't be given any more visas that season.

I exhaled with grateful relief. A change in plans I could deal with. "Don't say it's bad news unless someone died!" I joked.

The change meant that climbing from Tibet was out, so Pasang and I decided we would climb the route in front of us, on the south side of Everest. We were here and that was all that we could do, so we might as well enjoy it.

That night, I fell into a restless high-altitude sleep. I woke up every hour, hoping that when I opened my eyes the first light of dawn would have arrived. When it finally did, it came with the distant clamor of voices on the radio. I peeked out of my tent to see Dawa waving his hands and frantically motioning me to come up to his tent. I put on my down jacket and boots and headed up, unsure what the urgency was about.

"Meli, there was an accident. A big one. All Sherpas." He paused and I watched his Adam's apple bob as he attempted to swallow. "Many are dead." The words hung in space until he loudly exhaled. "Can you go up? They need help."

I took a breath to calm the flood of adrenaline that rose within me. Of course I would go. I assumed the familiar role of responder that I had practiced in my medical work, calm and intentional with my movement.

I hastily departed to get dressed, planning to climb up to the accident site and help however I could. I didn't have a harness or crampons, so I borrowed them from another climber and went straight to the helipad at the edge of camp, where all the rescuers had assembled. Since I had significant medical training and experience, it was quickly decided that I would fly up first with medical equipment. No one was totally sure what had happened at the accident site, but what little news we had was grim. A large number of local workers had been climbing together when the avalanche came swiftly down on top of them. Some were dead. Some were missing. And some were injured and desperate for care.

I boarded the helicopter, and a moment later we left solid ground and headed into something unimaginable. Tragedy was not new, nor was my facing it. Nearly every season that I had worked on Everest had included some sort of rescue or an up-close view of a tragic accidental death. That was part of the deal with the biggest mountains in the world. But I had never seen, nor even imagined, death on this scale. I had no time to wonder what it would be like—I just went in, closing my heart to the truth of what was in front of me and doing the job I was asked to do. Like so many times before, I knew I needed to seal off my emotions and do the task at hand. I could sort through the tragedy of it all later, and I would.

April 18, 2014

The air feels whisper thin and unoccupied. I stop, holding my own breath to see what I can hear. Nothing. Not a crack, nor a creak. Not even the sound of stillness. Here, everything is gone. Life is gone. It is as though something or someone has pressed pause on this moment in time and I am somehow allowed to look around and feel the absence of everything. Newton said that energy cannot be created or destroyed; it can only be transferred or changed from one form to another. I have felt that transfer many times, something turning into something else with the flip of a switch. But I wonder if Newton ever dreamed of something like this, a place where the earth opens and absorbs all the energy, leaving no trace of it behind.

The borrowed crampons on my feet are heavy and unfamiliar. But they talk to the glacier ice in the same familiar conversation of crunching and piercing, offering some comfort. I am at almost 20,000 feet and my lungs are burning like structure fires, telling me to slow down. The sound of my breath and the booming of blood flow is filling my ears now like the white noise of an ocean in chaos. It is not rhythmic. It is not peaceful. I move quickly, following the chucks of broken ice and the splashes of red blood that are smattered about. A backpack rests near a crimson stain in the snow. I don't know who it belongs to. I wonder if he lived or died. I keep moving, up and then down, covering every inch of the area in search of something missed. I am both eager to find something and dreading what it will be. And then, I see him. Upside down, suspended by the rope and the universe. Stopped right there and buried partially under hundreds of pounds of ice; entombed. I stop, allowing my breath to ease enough to speak. Keying the mic on the radio, I relay the news that I have found another one. We need to go check it out. The other rescuers rush from behind me, climbing up the slight incline around giant crevasses and blocks of ice, and continue to the broken battlefield ahead. I stay where I am, watching over them. I feel the weight of what might happen next pulling at us all. It feels like the mountain has only partially exhaled, and there is more to come. I do not want to be caught in her breath or see another life absorbed into her flanks. I will my soul to communicate with hers as I scour the slopes for any sign of movement. A helicopter lands below me and I see another body wrapped tightly, small and lifeless. It is loaded in and flown away. It is wrong to be seeing death on this scale. Stacks of bodies, ponds of blood, wails of loss. This is the stuff of war. This is for people who signed up for the possibility of carnage and had a moment to decide how they would handle it. But as that thought floats through, another comes to rest. Carnage is about the element of surprise. It is about accepting small losses over and over until one day you are faced with a loss you cannot ignore. A loss of size and scale you could not have even imagined.

Within a few hours, the final body has been freed from its icy tomb and wrapped and laid next to the others, waiting its turn to be loaded into the helicopter. We climb in and for a moment I feel a small sprig of gratitude that we are alive. Then I feel guilty and selfish for feeling anything good.

As we reintroduce ourselves to the rest of Base Camp, we cannot be understood. We are new people now. The others want to know what we saw. They want to feel grateful, too, that it was not them. But what can be said about death on this scale?

The Tibetans believe that a goddess lives inside every mountain. The one inside Everest is called Myosangmalangma, and she is extraordinary. She is fierce and powerful, riding on top of a wild white tiger that she has tamed. She is generous, holding a mongoose that spits gold coins and a basket of fruit that she willingly shares. She is different from the goddess that they believe resides in K2, Takar Dolsangma. That goddess is angry and has the taste for human flesh, which she will take to satiate her hunger. But not Myosangmalangma. If she takes a life, it is not for hunger, it is to teach you something. I wonder if I will learn the lesson she is offering. I wonder if I even can.

As night falls on the end of this horrific day, I look up at her moonlit flanks. She has taken so much, but she is quiet now. I do not feel anger toward her. I wonder what she is trying to say. I can feel her protective qualities, casting out over us all again, even amidst this great loss. I can sense her generosity still dormant under the veneer of terror she has cast. I silently make her a promise that I will listen. I am paying attention. With a settling crack, the icefall adjusts its position once more. I feel the vibration under my feet, and I feel her exhale in my soul. I breathe a deep breath, letting the air absorb into my body and exhaling gratitude back to her.

* * *

The details of the accident became more and more tragic as we pieced them back together. The Sherpas had been climbing up in the early hours of the previous morning when they arrived at one of the metal ladders that were placed to help cross the gaping crevasses. It was broken, making the route impassable, and they shed their loads to wait for the icefall doctors to come fix it.* They pulled out their thermoses and cigarettes and snacks and huddled together in a sort of dogpile to stay warm. A thunderous crack ripped through the sky. Two thousand feet above, an ice block the size of a suburban house calved off the cliff and careened down, breaking apart and spewing destruction in every direction. The men were buried. Those who tried to run were hit by ice chunks or knocked into crevasses hundreds of feet deep. The seven men who stayed huddled were crushed under the ice and under one another and mostly suffocated.

It was a tragedy that would affect every village in some way and bring the climbing season to a halt. Workers demanded a better safety net for their families if they were going to do such a dangerous job. Women in villages threatened to bring all the children and leave them at Base Camp if their husbands climbed. I sat with Pasang as we both cried. She had lost an uncle and knew almost every one of the sixteen who died. I knew six of them well after years of working alongside them on this very mountain. One was Ang Tshering, the Camp Two cook who had so tenderly helped me after Chhewang died.

I wondered how things might have been different for us if Pasang and I had our climbing gear. Would we have been caught too? I chose not to dwell on this what-if and instead decided to return home.

I stayed in Nepal for a week after we returned from the mountains to Kathmandu. I cried every day and felt empty and helpless. My sleep was interrupted by images of the ice splattered with blood. I would wake up wanting to flee from myself but with nowhere to go. By the time I got home to Idaho, I had placed all my feelings on a shelf with a label

---

* The icefall doctors are a group of Sherpas who are paid by every team to set the ropes and ladders in the icefall only. They don't go above Camp Two but instead work to keep the ever-changing route passable.

"Things No One Can Understand" and met everyone with quietness. I had spent a huge part of my adult life facing traumas on the ambulance and in the mountains, but this was on a scale that was much harder to wrestle down in my mind and soul. With Jon, I was icy, distant. I didn't even attempt to let him close. His best friend was getting married that May and he was excited that I could join him at the wedding now that I was back early. I resented his excitement and looked at him with disgust that he could find a bright side to something so horrific.

Truthfully, he didn't know what to do. Who would? He offered me all the space I needed but I greedily took more, wanting to be surrounded by only my own thoughts. I decided to ride my bike alone across Montana instead of going to the wedding, replacing one discomfort for another in the rhythm of survival that had brought me here. I started to seriously wonder if *here* was where I even wanted to be. How long would I be able to avoid the truth that was crashing down around me, a serac of its own?

17.

PEAK PURITY

2014: Mustang, Nepal

The blank slope of firm white snow the consistency of Styrofoam sprawled above me into the unknown. I looked down at Ben, his ice tools touching the ice and snow in front of him. The slope was steep enough that all he had to do was lean gently forward, as though smelling a pot of simmering soup, and his upper body would be inches from the surface. His red helmet contrasted with his yellow jacket and for a moment I thought he looked like a hot dog. Our teammate and photographer, Jon,[*] was on the slope to my right, looking for an easier way to ascend.

I took a deep breath, absorbing the tiny oxygen molecules at 20,000 feet above sea level and begging them to wash me clean. Just a short distance above me was the summit of this unclimbed peak, sprinkled

---

[*] Not my husband, a different Jon.

with loose rocks and frozen white ice, as pure as a virgin bride. I had long forgotten what purity even looked like, and when I saw it now in this mountain, it made me feel dirty.

We had spent the previous weeks exploring the unmapped zone of northwestern Nepal, looking for a trio of peaks that had only recently been opened by the government for climbing. I wanted to find mountains that were challenging but that would possibly allow someone with mediocre climbing skills to ascend them, not just so I could bring clients, but also to have an adventure that wasn't life-threatening. Basically, I was looking for a steep walk in a remote place. And now, after three days spent up high, we had found it. I was going to complete a first ascent of an unclimbed peak.

I felt giddy with the excitement of knowing that it was unlikely humans had stood here before. I imagined what it was like for the British mountaineers from the 1920s, and I almost wished I had brought a flag to plant. Of course, I wasn't here out of some sense of patriotism or exploration, but rather a sense of escape. And the kind of escape I was looking for required going deep into unmapped terrain, free from humans other than my small team. It required nearly getting lost on the Tibetan tundra to see if I could catch a glimpse of myself.

The death and the tragedy from the previous seasons were weighing heavily on me, reminding me how finite this life is. It was forcing me to look at my own choices and ask myself if I wanted to live my life pretending to be someone I wasn't or if I wanted to be truly known. I was hoping some time in the quiet of these mountains would help me find some answers.

The irony was that my career was rising for my suffering. I'd spent the last seven years on Everest in the spring, arriving at the summit five times. I spent every fall returning to the Himalayas, deepening my connection with the people, and sharing trekking peaks with clients. When winters arrived, I began a rigorous training regimen and took multiple trips to New York City to meet with the media and tell them how I was exceptional and interesting and worth keeping their eye on. I wrote a semi-honest essay in *Women's Health* about how marriage was my real Everest. I sat for filmed interviews with morning talk show hosts to discuss what it was like in the death zone, and more important, what it was like for a woman. The wave of success and attention was a steady and reliable swell, and I was surfing its every curve.

But at the same time, I was shrinking into a shell of a human. The only person I was anymore was the person the media saw, single-dimensioned and uncomplicated. Everything else was turning numb and dull, cloaked in dishonesty. I had kept cultivating my distance from my husband, and drinking in the attention of all the boys and men on expeditions. I was refusing every attempt at being a good partner, a good wife, or even a good person. The more I hid from myself and all that I was carrying, the more I sort of just disappeared into a mirage of the person the world saw.

When I was home, I couldn't even pretend to be present. I took an Ambien each night and drank too many beers, hoping the time would melt by and I wouldn't have to remember it. Jon worked during the day and played hockey and spent time with his friends instead of with me. He hated confrontation, so even if he wanted to bring up the distance, he didn't. I hid behind my training and my work. I slinked away on trip after trip to avoid him and the life I had pretended to choose. I wondered if Jon felt the space between us widening. I suspected he did.

By the fall of 2014, the cracks in our lives had opened to become man-gulping crevasses that no ladder could span. There was no more pretending to be close. There was nothing as simple as the touch of a hand or as deep as an embrace. There was just logistics. Did you walk the dog? When do I leave again? I wasn't just running away anymore; I was gone.

The autumn season started with my choice to arrive in Nepal ahead of my first group of clients to attend the Sherpa wedding of Cherap and Lhakpa's daughter Rhita, my Nepali "sister" to whom I had grown close over the past seven years. Jon wanted to go, but a college friend of his was getting married in Belgium at the same time, so we said goodbye and boarded planes going in opposite directions.

After Rhita's wedding, my client arrived and we trekked for three weeks, followed immediately by a second client and another three-week trek. These treks took us to the base of Everest but kept us on the hiking trail and far from the risks of climbing. I enjoyed seeing the mountain in this off-season; it was like visiting a friend. September and October came and went. I missed Jon's birthday and another friend's wedding back in Idaho. I asked a friend to bring a cake to Jon at our house, and when my friend told me a girl had answered the door, I felt nothing. I didn't feel like I had the right to care.

At the end of the second trek, my next climbing team arrived—my friend and climbing partner, Ben, and a photographer, Jon—and we began our expedition into the unknown. Sponsored by Eddie Bauer, we intended to tackle an unclimbed peak in the remote northwest border of Nepal and Tibet. The area was hard to reach, and thus tourists were scarce, making it alluring, exciting, and certainly an adventure. The farther we trekked into the valley, the less English was spoken or understood, and we had only vague maps to help us navigate toward the peak we intended to climb. This was going to be the longest time I had ever spent in Nepal. I left my home in Idaho in early September and I wouldn't return until after Thanksgiving. Jon and I chatted over WhatsApp only once a week, even less at times. I felt light and liberated, with no expectation to uphold my image and my life back home.

A few weeks into the expedition and just before noon, after days of climbing toward the unknown destination, we reached the summit of Mustang Himal, a 20,324-foot unclimbed peak on the border of China and Nepal. We hugged, took photos, and built a tiny cairn of stone to mark the summit. I slipped one of the red necklaces given to me by a high Lama, called a sungde, under the stone. We had done it. After the spring season on Everest had been interrupted by the tragedy of sixteen workers dying in the icefall, this climb felt redemptive, evidence that the mountains weren't only cruel. We descended back to civilization over the course of the next week, drinking Nepali lager at nearly every stop and celebrating our accomplishment. I wanted time to stop, suspended in a moment of good. A moment of truth. We were climbers. We were who we said we were, nothing to hide, which made the prospect of returning home to continue the lie all the more bleak.

The flight home was sleepless, despite another Ambien and too many drinks. My mind refused to quiet. Reckoning day was coming. I had to do something. I couldn't keep running away to Nepal. I couldn't keep lying to Jon while slipping further and further from the relationship I had promised to honor. If we were going to stay together, I was going to have to show up, truly and fully. I wanted to *want* to stay together, but that was as far as I had gotten in my assessing of what was next.

I stopped in Seattle on my way back to Idaho and had dinner with Christine after what had been a long season away. The darkness of November and the impending long winter ahead made me nervous, worried that the darkness would be too much on top of what was in my mind.

"I know marriage is hard. I just wonder . . ." I paused as I confessed my fears to Christine. "I just wonder if it is supposed to be this hard. Like sometimes I wonder if I am just not cut out to be a wife." My words hung in the room like a curse, but it felt good to finally just say it out loud.

"Marriage is hard," she comforted me. "You've had a hard few years. But I think you just have been gone for so long, it probably feels weird to go home. But once you do, it will all feel so much better." Her reassurances felt like what she thought she should tell me. She knew me, but she didn't know the truth. It wasn't the year behind, or even the one before, that was to blame. It was me. I had retreated, building a shield of armor before I ever said "I do." For all my desire to stay open, I had buckled at the fear of what openness risked: If I showed my true self to Jon, he could choose not to love me. But I had grossly misunderstood how lonely it was to hide behind a fortress of lies and deceit. And how much work it was. And how tired I would be.

I thought about how liberated Ueli had seemed as he put himself out there for all to see. His climbs were the ultimate act of vulnerability, risking everything, taking himself to the very limit physically and mentally. I could see that they were only possible because he maintained that vulnerability in his life as well. He was honest. He was who he said he was.

My desire to be honest was growing. I drove the ten hours from Seattle to Idaho, rehearsing my apologies to Jon. I wouldn't tell him everything, but I would admit that I hadn't been present. I hadn't given him a marriage. And I wanted that to change. I wanted to be partners again, and I wanted to try to be open to him again like I had in the earliest days of our relationship after Chhewang's death, when I was too tired to hold up a façade. As I drove, I wondered if being alone and with someone was better than being alone and alone. I wondered if the only reason I wanted to work on my marriage was because I feared failure and feared what other people would say about me. I shook the thoughts out of my head and reminded myself that I was going to fix this. I was not going to fail.

I walked into my house feeling like a stranger. Jon wasn't home. He had gone on a trip to Vegas because he wasn't expecting me back for a few more days. The house was cold and felt anonymous. We had no pictures on the walls; only metal art hung above concrete floors. I felt like it was what my own insides must look like. Our rooms were echoingly empty, making everything seem bigger than it really was, and making me feel somehow smaller.

I opened a bottle of wine and poured a glass. Jon's computer was on the counter, and I opened it, instinctively investigating who he was when I was gone. I opened his inbox and scrolled for notes that would make me feel better about my own deceit. I wanted the relief of knowing that I wasn't the only one who was imperfect. I looked at the open tabs on his browser and scrolled through them one by one. I opened his photos and suddenly my breath caught in my throat. Four photos. A girl in a cute selfie, taken from a car, smiling coyly. Her almost naked body spread over a white blanket with a stack of books in the corner. A lacy bra and the curves of her chest captured at just the right angle.

What had I been looking for? I wanted Jon to be as untrustworthy as I was, but now, confronted with nearly naked pictures of another girl, I felt like I was sinking. I felt myself gasping for air, trying to break free of the sense of betrayal pulling me under. The car in the photo had the steering wheel on the opposite side. The books in the corner were in Dutch. She was from Belgium. It took me forty-five seconds to find her on Facebook, and then to see their entire chat history. It took me ten more seconds to find his internet searches: "How to say love in Dutch," "Learn Dutch in 3 months." I picked up the wineglass, drank it all, and threw the glass down, shattering it on the concrete floor as tears and anger poured out of me.

I couldn't tell if I was madder at him or at myself. He wasn't supposed to have this power. I wasn't supposed to be hurt by him. What if he had told me as many lies as I had told him? My mind became a spiral stopped only by another bottle of wine and two Ambien. I hoped I would fall asleep. I didn't care if I woke up.

When Jon came home, I confronted him from the top of the stairs in the house that we had attempted to make our home. He froze when he saw me standing there, arms crossed and rigid. "I will give you one chance to tell me what is going on." My tone was even but direct, with the edges of a threat.

"Going on with what?" He slowly made his way up the stairs. I thought of my mom doing this same thing to me when I was a kid and how much I detested not knowing what I was in trouble for.

"Going on with you," I said, stepping aside as he passed me and walked toward the open computer with the images on the screen.

"This isn't what you think." His words were quick but my anger was quicker. I raised my voice and it bounced off the concrete floors.

"Get the fuck out of here. Leave!" I didn't allow him any chance to explain, and I didn't reveal any of my own truth or share the apology I had practiced on the drive.

In the weeks ahead, we fought and cried and negotiated. "Nothing happens in a vacuum." He said the words as we walked our dog across the open field near our home. "You haven't even touched my hand in months." I hated that he was telling me this was my fault. I hated that I knew he was right. He might have turned his attention on someone else, but I had done far worse.

I continued to hide behind my work and we agreed to get through the winter, me in the guest room and him upstairs. I was starting to film a six-part web series with *Glamour* magazine and *The Today Show*, chronicling my seventh season on Everest, and hopefully my sixth summit, this time without oxygen. I didn't have time for my marriage to fall apart, and Jon was happy to defer the inevitable, unaware that he wasn't the cause of our circumstances. We attempted counseling. Our therapist told me that wanting to climb at high altitude was a form of mental illness that needed to be treated separately for my marriage to ever work. I never went back to see her again.

* * *

After four months, when the time finally came to leave for Nepal again in the spring, I told myself I would deal with Jon, and my pain, when I got home. I just needed these months in this place I loved so much, to allow me to be ready.

It was early in the season and my small team had been working hard to capture the documentary footage for our partnership with *Glamour*. The photographer Jon and my climbing partner Ben from the previous fall were back on board, and we added Adam, a longtime friend, as a Base Camp manager and general helper.

But the feeling of freedom I had found in the mountains so many times before remained elusive. I couldn't escape the stress and pain, even there. The escape was no longer an escape; instead, it was acting as a magnifier of the contrast between who I wanted to be and who I was. My stress levels were peaking. I was creating mess after mess in my own life, and my normally enthusiastic self was starting to fade into anxiety and pain. I was pretending to be confident, unbothered, above it all, but the truth was, my heart was breaking, and breaking open. Up until now, I had been able to keep running away, changing my story, my life, my boyfriend, my identity. But now it was all settling on me. I had everything to lose, and it would be all my own fault.

I trudged through the depression that was slowly taking over my world and dimming all the vibrance to gray. I had a job to do, and I would do it. We set up our base camp and headed to a nearby peak to start the acclimatization process in earnest like I had so many seasons before. The weather so far had been as gray and moody as I felt, bringing monotones of silver and white with the snowstorms each afternoon. We climbed. Even the climbing felt like an act to me now, somewhat empty and lacking the presence I had always felt in the mountains. We slept in our little tent on the summit of the peak, just outside of base camp, and then descended to the village below for hot tea and to make a plan.

It was just after lunchtime on April 25 when we entered a small teahouse in Lobuche Village, just a two-hour walk from camp. I had spent countless nights in this warm and familiar teahouse, but on this day it felt cold and disconnected, just as I did.

I breathed deeply into my tea, smelling the pungent black leaves mingle with the sweet scent of sugar as I tried to pull myself out of the mind sludge. Suddenly the walls started shaking. A feeling pulsed through the center of my core, making me want to get up and run. It was an earthquake. A huge one.

Within seconds, everyone in the teahouse was pushing over one another to get outside as the walls and roof began to collapse. It was happening so fast, but I was seeing everything in slow motion. One piece of the roof fell in front of me, opening a hole to the snowy sky above. I looked up, wanting to escape out of that hole instead of standing in the chaotic wreckage all around. This teahouse, falling down as the earth vibrated, felt like what my heart must look like. Shaking, breaking, and changing forever. My team made it outside along with all the other people who were just as surprised as us. The walls of the building still stood, but the roof had fallen in. We could have been buried, but instead we stood looking at one another with a mix of confusion and elation at having survived. We had no connectivity to the outside world and for a moment it felt like this all might be a dream.

In the hours that followed the initial quake, we tried to determine how widespread the shock was, and if anyone was injured. Instead of returning to base camp we descended the valley to a lower village, hoping to be able to get news of what had happened.

The quake was far bigger than we could have imagined, 7.8 magnitude. Nepal had been devastated. Thousands of people had died in Kathmandu and the villages surrounding the mountains. Homes were leveled, and entire villages were covered by mudslides. At Everest Base Camp a catastrophic air blast* had hit the camp like a hurricane. Whole camps were picked up and moved two hundred feet or more. Nineteen people died, and others suffered head injuries, lost limbs, and trauma from the force of flying rocks, ice, and objects.

All the expeditions ended before they began. We stayed for some days at base camp, cleaning up what was left of our camp and expedition, but as soon as it was safe we headed for the stable ground of our homes. Of course, my home and life were in an upheaval of their own. I didn't even want to return. I was feeling lonelier than I ever thought possible as my daily existence grew more suffused with darkness. I saw Jon and felt nothing. I knew it had ended, but even the finality of that thought could barely force out a tear. I felt empty and turned inside out in a way I hadn't felt since I was a teenager sitting on my parents' porch swing. I had thought the previous fall, when I returned home to Jon's deceit, must be the bottom. But the bottom kept sliding, further and further, and now I was floating in the space of my own creation, a bottomless place, unanchored to real life. Nothing mattered because nothing was real.

---

* An air blast is a hurricane-force wind that can precede an avalanche, creating equal devastation.

* * *

It was spring and I wanted to ask Jon for a divorce, but instead decided to go on an expedition to the remote glaciers of east Alaska. Running was better than feeling. Motion numbed the intensity of stillness. And mountains had always been able to hide my truth. But now, as I tried to escape again, the escape was pushing me back toward my life at home and the inevitability of dealing with years of trying to be someone who seemed loved while refusing to be seen enough to *be* loved. I wanted all the riches with none of the risk, and my world was starting to crumble around me.

My small team from Everest had reunited in the hope of some healing and adventure after the trauma of the earthquake. We headed to Alaska, where we were dropped on a glacier by a small plane on skis, with the plan of being picked up in two weeks.

This expedition was supposed to be easy and fun. We should have planned a beach trip. The mountains, even when they are fairly benign, are always challenging. My successes over the years on Everest and other peaks had somewhat muted that knowledge in my brain. It seemed to me that things were either extremely straightforward or horrendously tragic. The truth was that most expeditions lived in the space between those two experiences. Alaska would, on this trip, remind me of that.

The journey started off like many before, with optimism and curiosity. But as we made our way up Mount Bear, our 14,829-foot heavily glaciated objective, our optimism was met with a swat of Mother Nature's paw. First the storms came. Then the navigation became grueling with team members falling into hidden crevasses and dangling over the abyss while the rest of the team hauled them out with elaborate rope rescue systems. Then, on the seventh day, we were almost out of fuel and the snow and clouds only strengthened. There would be no summit, and it was obvious we had to retreat to our base camp.

Eventually, we were scooped up in a plane and returned to the dusty runway and green grass of sea level. The time on the glacier had been meant to refill my soul and offer me some clarity, but instead I returned five pounds lighter and feeling emptier than ever. I called Christine from the sat phone while I was still in Alaska and told her to cancel all my work for the summer. She politely declined and told me to go get some food, and we could talk later.

But I didn't want there to be a later. I needed to go back to the house I shared with Jon and end things. I needed to find some sort of center and decide how to move forward. I needed to stop the downpour in my mind, as all the shameful things I had done in my whole life rained into any quiet space. But all those tasks felt as impossible as navigating a whiteout on a massive glacier. I didn't even know which way was up.

I was scheduled to fly to Tibet the next week to guide a trek, and so I returned to Idaho, intent on change. At ten a.m. on a Tuesday I texted Jon and asked if he could come to the house to talk to me. I sat at our dining room table on the beautiful wooden bench that he had built, bathed in the sun of a June morning. The birds tweeted joyfully, and the smell of a fresh-cut lawn seeped in through the screen door. I remembered how the smell of the grass used to make me feel the joyful hope of a summer spent in the mountains, but today the smell made me feel nauseated. I wrapped my legs in a crisscross twisted pretzel of protection, the same way I had learned from the mountain gods years before, guarding myself from being seen.

Jon came into the house timidly. We hadn't spoken much since I had returned from Nepal and Alaska. He stood while I sat. He looked tired, his eyes sunken and ringed with gray. I counted to three in my head, and at three I forced the words out of my mouth. "I want to get divorced." My words flopped out with no inflection. My head didn't move but my eyes looked up at him, unwavering in my plan. I wrapped my legs tighter, guarding myself more. I wouldn't let him hurt me.

He quickly turned and hit the wall beside him with his palm, causing a vibration and a smacking sound at the same time. This was a surprise to me, but I held as still as a statue, a skill I'd learned in childhood. Don't react to their reactions. I hadn't expected him to have this one.

His back was to me, which felt about right. I had turned my back on him, so I didn't deserve much more than that now. "You don't want to even try!" His words burst out, hitting me with the pressure of his exhale as he turned to face me. "I know you, and when you want something, you fight for it. You don't even want to try." His voice cracked with emotion.

He was right. I didn't want to try. My eyes gazed at him, dead and dark without even the smallest glisten of the emotion he was looking for. I told him I was going to Tibet and that we should think about the practical steps of separation—selling our house, dividing our things. I told him to let me know what he wanted and I would do the same. He took one final long look at me. There was disappointment in his eyes. It looked familiar. I had seen it before—I had practically lived my life around seeing it and fleeing it. The guilt of doing a bad thing would turn to the shame of being a bad thing, and from there all I could do was run.

He moved closer to me, and I wondered if he was going to try to hug me. He leaned forward so his face was just one inch from mine. I was still sitting on the bench and he stood, hunched over me now as though I were a child. I felt his breath escape gently as his words slipped out in a near whisper. "I gave you everything. You just wouldn't take it. Nothing is ever enough." And then he turned and left.

The door slammed shut and I covered my eyes with my hands and breathed in, trying to resist the tears that were catching in my throat. He was right. It wasn't that I had never been loved; he had loved me as fully and openly as I had let him, but I had never believed that love was truly meant for me, that I deserved it. As a result, his love seemed like a lie to me.

I pushed the tears back down and stood. I didn't have time to sit in this pain or try to solve the problem that I had become. I didn't want to solve it. And I had to pack for Tibet.

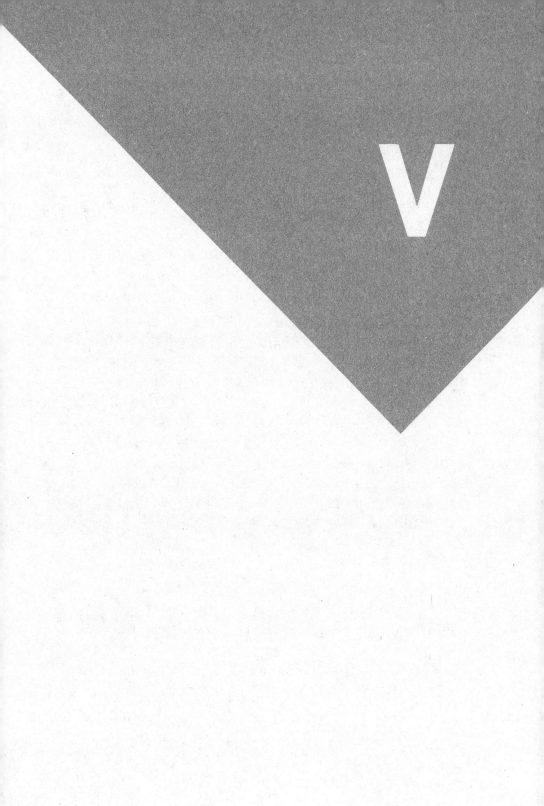

18.

LIBERATION

2015: Tibet, China

"*Om Tare Tuttare Ture Soha, Om Tare Tuttare Ture Soha, Om Tare Tut-tare Ture Soha . . .*"

Tiny droplets of dirty water flung off my flip-flops and onto the backs of my legs with each step. It was impossible to avoid the puddles from the buckets of water the monks were throwing to tamp down the dust around the monastery in Lhasa, the capital city of Tibet. The early-morning sunlight trickled gently through the heavy smoke of burning juniper. The smoke created a blanket hanging in the air around me for a moment before it floated up to the gods. The rhythmic sound of monks dropping their bodies onto the granite courtyards surrounding the holy site was both alarming and hypnotizing. Facing forward, hands overhead in a sort of sun-salutation prayer, they would then drop to their knees, hands holding the little blocks that reminded me of sand-paper holders. Then they would slide forward until their bodies lay flat on the dirty ground in a sort of Superman dive—showing reverence to the enlightenment contained within the monastery. Finally, they would complete the cycle by sliding back up to return to standing with a quiet Tibetan chant starting deep in their belly and seeping out their lips. This would go on for hours of days of their entire lives, the monks repeating the prostration 108 times in each session.

To see their weathered and aging bodies suggested that something might be gained through a commitment to discomfort, something discovered in the rhythms of standing and lying, breathing, and chanting.

I walked the meditative circle around the outside of the monastery, slowly and alone, in the mandatory clockwise direction. A complete circle of meditation, or a kora, as the Tibetans called it. I marked my journey each time I passed the front gate and met the smoky haze of the burning juniper.

I was in Tibet to fulfill a commitment I had made the previous year to guide a group of affluent yoga practitioners from Silicon Valley on a tour through the country. We would make our way to Everest Base Camp after viewing all the holy sites and historical villages along the way, the entire tour made by jeep and interrupted only for lessons about yoga in the mornings and Buddhism in the afternoons. After trying unsuccessfully to escape this obligation, and all the others I had committed to that summer, I was now just trying to be present.

Since I had asked Jon for a divorce, the days were blending into each other. I just wanted them all to go faster, but I couldn't escape the life I had created. I was no longer able to distract myself from the darkness. None of the beauty and nuance of Tibet, which I had been to before, could break through the dull indifference coating every part of my mind. What had started as a dimming of life's vibrance had turned full black, dark, numb, and frighteningly lonely. The mountains weren't fixing it. The travel wasn't fixing it. The bottle of wine I drank every night wasn't fixing it. When I looked inside myself, I saw the person I had been hiding from myself and others for years: someone who was truly not lovable. Not by me or anyone else.

My dirty and slightly wet feet kept shuffling around the monastery, making the koras. At the front gate for the eleventh time, I decided to enter. The ornate gold of the gates shone bright under a sun that was rising higher each minute. As I entered the monastery, my eyes took a moment to adjust to the dark interior. I was struck by the contrast with the building's bright façade, decorated lavishly with gold and shining symbols. A tightness formed in my throat as I recognized this contrast in myself. I wondered if I could ever love the dark interior of my own self as much as the worshippers loved this place.

That was when I saw her.

The room's dark walls were decorated with paintings of Buddhas and various gods and goddesses, but from across the space, on the wall farthest from the doorway, one of them caught my eye. It pulled me forward. The musty smell of a very old room that was frequently full of the sweaty bodies of monks pierced my nostrils as I crossed, and a moment later I was standing before her. She was a human-size painting hung in the darkest corner of this ancient building. I inched closer, feeling pulled by a horizontal gravity unlike anything I had felt before. Everything around looked muted and dingy, but she gave off a warm glow in hues of teal and jade. I looked up, expecting to find a light source or a skylight, but there was nothing. The green glow was coming directly from her. It felt like it was being cast into me. The hairs on my neck stood as I heard what sounded like a whisper. *Come closer.* I looked around, but no one was near me.

Over several years of traveling in Nepal, I had seen Buddhas and bodhisattvas and paintings of gods and goddesses too numerous to count. They made up the background fabric of a place I loved, and while each was beautiful and intricate and captivating, none had ever spoken *to* me. And here she was, ready to spring into action with her leg outstretched, calling me toward her with a mature but kind face. Suddenly my throat felt tighter, the kind of fullness you feel just before the tears. I was encapsulated in a soft, kind light as I approached her. The temperature of the room shifted. The old building had felt empty, cold, but now I seemed to be standing in front of a heater. She was casting warmth out. I could actually feel it.

The hairs on my arms and neck remained standing as I examined the painting closely. Her eyes seemed to drill into my center, to that place where I was hiding all my shame. She didn't look away. I felt her warmth envelop my entire body. I felt something I could describe only as acceptance. I inched close enough to her that I could feel her soft breath on my face. The tightness in my throat turned warm and fluid and I had the desire to simultaneously laugh and cry.

I bathed in her warm light for a few moments and then turned to leave, not wanting to be greedy with the moment. I wasn't sure if it was real, and the sudden burst of emotion and color was jarring after having felt so empty for so long. As I walked away, my breath was caught in my chest, making me feel lightheaded. I had lived a life of deeply tangible experiences, and this was like nothing I had seen or felt before. It was divine and strange.

I returned to the courtyard where the rest of the group was doing yoga and found Gary, one of the other leaders. A former lawyer turned Zen Buddhist and an expert in world religions, Gary had oversize glasses that would slip slowly down his nose as he spoke, and he always had a big camera dangling from his neck. He often got separated from the group and we would find him wandering toward some curiosity that had escaped everyone else's view. I liked him, and I found his teachings to be simple and easy to understand.

"Gary, can I ask you about one of the paintings I saw in the monastery? There was a Buddha but different from the standard seated one. I feel like it was a goddess of some sort, with a glowing green light all around her. I have never seen anything like it." I tried to ask without revealing that I might be having a mental breakdown.

"Of course!" he replied. "Green Tara! She is exceptional and different from all the other Buddhas. She is actually considered the mother of them all. She is the reincarnate of a princess in Nepal, so it's surprising you haven't seen her before." He paused and pushed his glasses up his nose. "She is mature and gentle and available to help you develop your inner qualities and understand your outer ones, like a mother. Very loving." Like nearly all the symbols in Buddhism, he explained, she was there to free you from suffering. She was not just a mother but the mother of liberation.

The Tibetan sun shone hot overhead as we spoke. I watched Gary's glasses sliding farther down his nose, thinking that I hadn't known a mother to be loving. What I did know was that the Green Tara had reached out directly to me. I wanted to tell Gary all about it, but I wasn't sure how he would respond, so I kept it to myself. Instead, over the next few days, I read all I could find about her. For the rest of the trip, each time I stumbled onto an incarnation of her, I stood near it feeling that same drenching warmth of acceptance. She could see me, all the way into my broken heart, and she doused me with the warm light of love anyway. I wondered if she was doing this for everyone, or if she was committed to setting me free.

* * *

The trip went on without any more paintings talking to me. I walked hundreds of circles around the dusty monasteries of Tibet and taught the clients how to breathe on the high-altitude tundra of Everest Base Camp. I drank too much wine, still dreading heading home to a full summer of guiding in the Cascades and Colorado. But, once again, home wouldn't wait, and as I returned from Tibet, I felt exhausted from the jet lag and my own unquiet mind. After so many attempts to run away from myself, it was starting to become clear that I truly could not escape what I was carrying inside me—I could only delay facing it, and the delays were becoming exhausting.

I had a week to get myself straight before working again, and I decided to pilgrim back to a geographic place of joy. I was hopeful that the landscape and my past with it could somehow rinse out the negativity I was carrying and give me a chance to look closer at why my world looked and felt as it did. I was craving the aloneness of the mountains not so much as a retreat from myself, but in a way, a retreat back to myself.

I packed the truck and headed to Montana. As I arrived in Bozeman, the sun was setting low on the horizon, cradled by the beautiful mountains that had cradled me so many times in my early days of learning how to climb and be a climber. The light cast a yellow-orange glow, and as it hit me it felt familiar and yet different. After the months of sadness and hurt and attempts to escape my own mind, this light felt supple and soft and kind. Instead of the soft orange of an early-summer sunset in the mountains, it felt warm and penetrating, like the light cast out of the Green Tara in Tibet. It felt like a beginning, not an end.

I made my way to an anonymous Hampton Inn situated on a busy street in a town I no longer recognized after so much time away. It was where I had landed when I first returned to Montana after my stint in Iowa, the place where I started to see myself as someone who belonged in the mountains. So much had changed in this town since I last lived here. I had changed, too. But the room was predictable and neutral, and that felt good.

I looked at myself in the bathroom mirror for the first time in a long time. Dark eyes, wet and ready to pour out tears at any moment. The creases of tortured decisions and the tragedy of the past years showing deep on my forehead. The freckled nose of so many days under the high-altitude sun. I rubbed my hands over my face, smoothing the skin between my eyebrows and closing my eyes. Since Tibet, little gaps of light had started to seep into my world. I laughed at a joke; I asked a friend to have dinner. I had gotten a handhold on the edge of the darkness, but knew I wasn't out of danger; I could easily fall deeper in. I drank wine alone in the room, then lay down.

As wakefulness faded to sleep, my consciousness became wrapped in the gentle green-blue light of a transition. I was not quite fully asleep, but in the space just between sleep and waking where your body sometimes startles with a little jump. And in that space, I could feel that I wasn't alone.

It was the Green Tara. She was here. Her feet were completely silent as she moved through the room. My eyes stayed closed, watching this dream but knowing that I was somewhat awake. Her head was turned slightly to one side and her fingers intertwined with one another as she approached me. I lay completely still in the bed, holding my breath, not opening my eyes for fear either that she would disappear or that she might actually be in the room, both frightening prospects. She stroked my hair and rubbed her long fingers over my forehead, leaving a green glow to everything she touched. I could feel the warmth on my own face where her hands had been. There was an ethereal gentleness that accompanied her every move. I couldn't help but notice the relaxed half-smile on her lips—not joy, but more the slight upward curve of contentment.

I fell deeper into a dream state and further from reality, but she journeyed with me. Suddenly, and without the same tenderness of her previous moves, she cut open my chest in a hexagonal shape and pulled out a heap of dark black matter. I looked at it, relieved to know that I had been right: My inside was as dark as I thought it was. I watched her closely, expecting her to cast it aside, cast me aside. But she embraced the dark matter lovingly. She sprinkled it into the air and it dissipated into a vapor like the smoke of burning juniper. I saw it change form from something dark and heavy into something white and weightless. My eyes followed her through the room until she settled herself into a seated position, legs crossed. Her hand touched her own chest above her heart, and she was gone. I touched the spot on my chest that she had opened and it was soft and warm and full of a sweet bouquet of wildflowers, pouring out and filling the bed around me. The darkness had been replaced by the growth and abundance of something wild and beautiful.

I woke up the next morning, the Fourth of July. The room was the same but the world felt completely different to me. I lay on the bed surrounded by soft blankets and pillows and enjoyed the sensation of comfort. I hadn't felt it in so long. Blinking my eyes, I looked up at the white ceiling, replaying the dream from the night before. I had seen my own darkness pulled from deep within me, incapable of being hidden any longer. As I visualized the dark gooeyness, I breathed slowly and deeply, in and out. I had a new feeling suddenly and clearly in my heart: I could let my darkness go. I could stop living with the shame of the belief that I was unlovable. I had seen my inner darkness treated with kindness and love and then let go. The Green Tara was a goddess, and if she could confront my darkest self with love, couldn't I do the same?

I stayed in the bed for a long time, eyes closed as I imagined five-year-old Melissa, feeling overlooked. I went to her, held her, and told her she was loved. I watched twelve-year-old Melissa, eager to be accepted and wanted as she fell in love with an adult man who would harm her. I told her I forgave her; it wasn't her fault. I visited twenty- and twenty-eight- and thirty-one-year-old Melissa and told her that she was in fact enough. My hand lay gently over my chest, not hiding my heart anymore, but holding it. And with each visit to my former self, I tried to give myself the same grace the Green Tara had in my dream.

I returned to the mirror and looked at my own eyes again. They were lighter. My soul was lighter, almost rising out of my body. My shoulders opened and my chest came forward. I saw a person who deserved to hurt but also deserved to move on. I had emptied my entire self out, and looked deep inside to see what was left. The destruction of my pain felt sudden, but really it had taken years. It had taken seven seasons on Everest, multiple failed relationships, a divorce, and an estrangement from my parents. Once I was finally, truly alone, I couldn't hide behind the perpetual motion or the illusion of who was to blame. It was me. To have love, I would first have to give love. I had to love myself, flaws and imperfections and all. I had to forgive myself. This revelation stole my breath. This pain was done teaching me. It was time to let it go. I saw myself through the compassionate eyes of the Green Tara. I knew I could be free.

* * *

That day was new. The air was clearer, the sun warmer. It felt like I was standing on the summit, and all the possibilities were in front of me again. I knew that it was going to be okay. I knew that I could heal and I didn't have to keep hiding. The darkness was leaving as the glow of acceptance grew.

I hiked deep into the mountains that morning and swam in the cold water of an alpine lake. As I pushed uphill under the warm July sun, I felt whole for the first time in a long time. Movement felt like a reward instead of punishment. I knew that I had a hard road ahead, that nothing could be solved overnight. There would be pain and difficulty. I would have more discomfort to face in my life. I would have to deal with the logistics of divorce, selling my house and starting over. But inside that I could feel the space of possibility. The hours spent in the bed that morning forgiving and loving my former selves felt like the first step in allowing anyone in. I needed to stop being ashamed. I had made mistakes, but I had also survived so much, and I deserved to heal and live. I felt a little smile of contentment settle onto my lips.

19.

MANIFEST

2015: Mount Rainier, Washington

The flanks of Mount Rainier stretched out in front of me in the evening twilight. A calm pink glow covered everything as the sun settled in. I stepped rhythmically, setting the pace for Ellie. She had started doing some mountain mentorship with me at the request of her parents, and now she was deep in her first glacier adventure as we tried to climb Rainier. She was quiet, but ambitious and driven. She was twelve years old, and spending time with her brought me back to my own twelve-year-old self and thoughts of how very different my life might have been. I didn't know a thing about climbing or even camping at that age, but I did know about survival. Sharing this space with Ellie felt curious and also healing, as I was starting the journey of living my life in a more open and vulnerable way. There was nothing quite like spending time with a pre-teen's blunt curiosity to let you know what you might still be hiding.

We had sat out a couple of storm days in Ashford, the small town at the base of Rainier, leaving us with only one choice if she wanted to try to summit that summer: climb in a single push from the parking lot at 5,400 feet all the way to the summit and back down in a day. I had climbed this way a few times and it was always an intense endurance challenge. Ellie was strong, and I was excited to see her challenge herself, so we moved steadily uphill.

A week had passed since my awakening in Montana, three since I had left Tibet. A month and a half ago I had asked Jon for a divorce. But it had been years since I had felt this good. I felt centered for the first time since my earliest days working on Rainier. A sense of belonging was slowly emerging from somewhere deep inside. It felt as though I had been reading a book upside down for my whole life and someone, the Green Tara perhaps, had come and flipped it right side up. Suddenly I could see how hard I had been making things and how easy they might be if I had been able to drop my guard and accept help far sooner. I had been attempting to do everything in my life all by myself. But the cracks that had opened up in the weeks and years behind me were starting to reveal that the person inside was strong, not weak. I was slowly able to see why I had been protecting myself, and I was finally able to begin to forgive myself for the mistakes I had made. I had started counseling again and was tending to my inner wounds rather than just running away and pretending I was okay.

As darkness surrounded Ellie and me and we made our way above 10,000 feet, the mountain provided us with the challenges we had come for. The terse wind in the cold night reminded me that I had chosen this challenge. I would survive the discomfort. There was much more of it ahead, I imagined. Deciding where I would live. Deciding to be fully myself and not pretending to be someone else. Healing the friendships that I had pushed away. Healing my relationship with my parents and my sister. Healing my relationship with myself. All of this would be discomfort, but I would stay. I would let the hurt grow me. I wouldn't run toward another pain but stay with this one until it was complete and the pain floated away like the darkness the Green Tara had pulled from inside me.

Night settled onto us along with the cold at 12,000 feet on the upper mountain. "How you doing, Ellie?" I glanced back at her petite frame, barely bridging the gap between childhood and teen years. The wind was chapping her face and her cheeks were cherry red. Her hat was slightly too big and kept creeping over her eyes.

She pushed it up with a gloved hand and looked up at me. "This is amazing!" She had spoken so few words that it was hard for me to gauge what was going through her mind. But the tone in her voice revealed that she was here, present and soaking it all in. I smiled, knowing this experience was going to change her in some way. That was the magic of the mountains when you showed yourself to them; they would reflect back all the possibilities of who you could be. My crampons pierced the firm glacier in the same way they had for the last ten years. This mountain had taught me how to move quickly and how to stay still. This mountain had shown me how strong I was, especially when I pushed myself to be open and vulnerable. The sunrise started to push the night away, and again, a pink glow coated everything. Ellie was doing great. We would get to the top in a few hours. I was glancing at her, watching her move and grow before my very eyes.

I could see the guides of RMI ahead of me and I wondered who it might be. I still had many friends and acquaintances there, but across the years the ranks had been replenished with people I had never met. Peter Whittaker had left Eddie Bauer the year before and started his own outerwear company, which further distanced our relationship. I hardly ever saw him, and now that I was going to leave Sun Valley, I knew that we would interact even less. But that felt okay, too. He had shared so much with me and shown me how to get the things I wanted most—to be a lead guide and work on Everest and have sponsorship and recognition. But I knew I needed more than just that external validation. I wanted connection and closeness. I wanted to be truly known and to know the people in my life beyond assessing what they could do for me. There was a tender space inside me that needed to emerge, to be seen and grow.

My mind wandered to all the guides I had worked with through all the years. I thought about Tyler, the new guide who was my assistant right after my first Everest climb in 2008, and how he had gracefully listened to me answer question after question, and feigned interest though he knew the story of my summit well. He had started his own guide service with his wife, and I wondered if he was still also guiding for RMI. I hoped I wouldn't run into my ex-boyfriend Brad. I thought about some of the mountain gods who had shown me how to get clients up and down and how to rig complex rescue systems. I didn't feel like one of them anymore, and that felt somewhat good, though I remembered the feeling of wanting so badly to be just like them.

As I shared my experiences with Ellie, a mountain mentorship began to form. It wasn't about testing her and breaking her down and making her prove something. That was the way I had been taught, but this was different. This was meant to be nurturing and curious. This was the way of the Mountain Goddesses, I thought. This was the way a mother would share her gifts. A mother goddess. I smirked just considering that I could be one, though I knew I had so much to learn to get there.

At just after eight a.m., as the sun drenched us with the warmth of a July morning, Ellie and I topped out on Rainier. The wind was calm, and the glacier was reflecting her radiance on us. I was so proud of Ellie, climbing continuously for fourteen hours to get there. As we crossed the snow-covered volcanic crater, we passed the mountain gods and their clients. I said hi to all the boys who looked the same and kept moving until one shouted at me. "Is that Melissa?" His words were muffled behind the thin fabric of the gaiter covering his mouth.

"Who's that?" I replied, shielding the sun from my eyes as I tried to determine if it was someone I knew. And it was. It was Tyler!

I gave him a hug and told him that I was just thinking about him. "Maybe I manifested you!" I exclaimed, thrilled to see his friendly face again.

"Can you do that?!" He laughed back at me.

"I just did!" I said. I told him how strong Ellie was, and that it was good to see him again. Then we coiled our ropes and parted ways for the descent. But he stayed in my mind as I climbed. I wondered about co-incidences and energy, and if I somehow had sensed he was there and that was what brought him to the front of my memories. I had worked with hundreds of guides over the years, and I wondered why it had been Tyler that had surfaced in my mind, ahead of all the rest.

I drove Ellie to the airport the next morning and headed back to Rainier to guide another climb. It felt good to be migrating back to the simple summit climbs with which I'd started my career. I was glad I hadn't canceled my whole summer schedule like I'd wanted to after Alaska. So much had changed in that short time, and it felt nice to settle into the simple rhythm of my season. As I sat in the morning meeting surrounded by mostly guides I didn't know, Tyler walked in. He made a comment to me about my being too much of a celebrity to guide here now, and I made a face at him. That afternoon, after we had ascended the snowfield with our clients and tucked them in to rest before the climb commenced at midnight, we sat on the rocks of Camp Muir, re-connecting.

In 2008, when I met Tyler, he had just been hired as a new guide, along with his girlfriend, Katy. They were both kind and quiet. They shared an old white Subaru Outback that carried surfboards and paddle-boards, defining them as adventurous coastal people. Tyler was my as-sistant guide on climb after climb, and we laughed that we were paired so frequently. I wasn't typically allowed to be friends with any male guides without Brad's blessing, but Tyler didn't even catch his eye. He wasn't an alpha. He was in a committed relationship.

Tyler and Katy faced all the challenges of being a couple in this bru-tal new industry. After they had survived their first year, she quit guiding and they eventually got married. Seven years went by. Tyler started his own guide service, focusing on skiing and the Olympic Mountains on the Washington coast. I hadn't seen him for years. I asked him how Katy was, and he told me unceremoniously that they were getting divorced. I felt curiosity spread over me as I told him I was getting divorced as well, and we agreed to drink a cocktail and share our stories, seeing if they intersected in any secret languages. I hadn't told anyone that I was getting divorced from Jon, even though we had been separated for almost a year. Saying it felt surprisingly good, like I was finally free. Like I wasn't existing in the in-between and unknown anymore. Like *I* wasn't unknown anymore. I was holding myself to the commitment I had made to be open even when I feared it made me look weak, even if I felt weak.

After that climb, a few weeks passed before I made time to meet Tyler for a drink. He had a calm confidence and a peaceful soul, and mine leapt out to meet it. His ease reminded me of my father. I was curious in a way I had never been before. I was seeing him as a person, much like me, with flaws and strengths and the potential to love and be loved. After years of pairing myself with people based on what they could do for me without ever fully opening up to them, I wasn't used to seeing anyone this way.

We spent the night on the porch of my cabin at the base of Rainier, talking and laughing and sharing things that only two thirty-year-olds going through divorce could share. "The year that Chhewang died . . ." I told him, slowly opening up, "that was the year that everything started to fall apart for me. I felt so broken that I just wanted to pretend I was whole and ignore all that pain." I was finally sharing out loud that I wasn't impenetrable, that the traumas in my life were sinking in and I had merely been doing my best to fight them off for all these years.

As I shared my feelings of shame, Tyler nodded, listening intently. "You aren't a *bad* person," he said. "You are just a person." He whispered these words, gently giving me permission to be honest with him. Our conversation continued the dance between heavy and light as we got to know each other, and the hours raced by in a blink. As I hugged him goodbye at three in the morning, we promised to meet up again soon.

I felt the stir of something I had never even believed in. There was nothing to gain from a relationship with Tyler. There was no equation of advancement like the ones that had been applied to each of my relationships before. He was him, and I was me, and together we formed a little buzz of energy that felt like perfect pitch, or a scale in tender balance. I had been holding back so much of myself for fear of being rejected for my flaws, but in one evening I had been able to open up more to him than I had in my entire relationship with Jon.

I lay awake that night, wondering what soulmates really were. Tyler couldn't be my soulmate. He was a surfer, a skier, and he had an obsessive love of reggae music. He had his own life and his own scars, and both of those diverged from mine. But the flutter of curiosity was unavoidable.

I fell into a semi-lucid dream state. Tyler was there, and we were starting a life together. I soaked in the feeling as the dream continued. When I woke, I couldn't fully comprehend the emotions and thoughts I was having, but I wanted to continue to bask in the glow of this new dream that might be possible. I didn't want to jump quickly into another relationship, but this felt like something completely different. *I* felt different. The premise of our connection had been formed in the vulnerability of openness. Turning away from Tyler now would be the easier thing to do, but I wanted to stay. I wanted change in my life, and this was the start of living in a new world where I didn't calculate my next move but instead stayed present and felt all the things, moving forward with a sense of wholeness that I had been missing for nearly my whole life.

I met him again the next day, and after we kissed and shared an exchange of vulnerability, I asked him if he knew what love was. "I used to," he said, sadness in his voice. He had had his heart broken. The pain was still fresh. It made him question so much of what he thought he knew.

I pushed him further. "What about the love of a friend? Or your mom?" He had shared stories of his closeness with his mom and how they enjoyed making music together.

"Well, yes. That love. I do know what that love is." He seemed unsure of where this question was going.

"Well, so do I," I told him, as he held me in his arms. "And I love you," I said. I was resisting my urge to moderate my thoughts and calculate my actions. I whispered the words, feeling something within me crumbling. This was a huge risk. This was a messy bundle of inconvenient emotions. I had no way to know where it would go or how he might feel as we learned more about each other. But the feeling was all-encompassing, and I had promised myself I would be rigorous in sharing what was really in my heart. I had spent so much of my life protecting my real feelings from showing, and here I was, outing myself and just being willing to go where it would take us.

* * *

In the months that followed we opened our schedules and hearts to each other, slowly finding footing on ground that had felt very uncertain just months ago. He lived in Washington and was in the process of separating his life from his ex-wife's while I did the same with Jon. We had divorced but the house wasn't sold yet, so we traded time there, interacting in a limited way. I told Jon about Tyler and told him that I thought it was an important relationship. He wanted to know if I had interacted with Tyler at all while we were married, and I told him no. I didn't have the courage to tell him any more than that, but I was honest about Tyler.

I drove to Washington, and Tyler and I spent our days off sitting by the ocean, eating avocados and sharing in the warm glow of new love. "Let's go on an adventure," he said as he packed a small backpack early one morning. We hiked up the hills around his house, the ones he had grown up in, and basked in the closeness we felt. We made space and time to talk about the hard things; he continued to heal from the end of his marriage, and I shared with him the story of my childhood. He held my truth with tenderness and asked questions about how it felt to me now. It hurt, now, to look back at the acceptance I had craved as a child and know that I didn't get it. But it also felt powerful to share that with another person. I had never admitted out loud that it was something I still craved, for fear of seeming weak. But with him I felt safe, at my best or my worst.

As our relationship progressed, I knew he would need to meet my parents. I had been keeping my distance from them since I told them that Jon and I were divorcing. I feared that they would want to talk about it, or blame me, and I couldn't handle that.

"What if you do something completely different with them?" Tyler asked. "What if you ask them to come to Idaho and stay with you?" He cared deeply about my past pain, but also about the possibility of healing it by closing the distance I had held for so many years. The thought made my body feel stiff, the instinctual protective posture I had held since I was a child. But he was right. If I wanted things to be different, and I did, I needed to be willing to try.

My parents accepted my invitation and spent a weekend in Idaho with Tyler and me. I felt the familiar anxious tension that I had grown used to when they were around, but I promised myself that I would try to allow things to be different. I had spent years fearing that they were only seeing me as the child who hurt them, refusing to see that I had grown and changed. But the truth was, I was holding on to the view of them as the parents who hurt me. I wasn't allowing them to be anything more from my perspective, and every action and word was filtered through the lens of the child I had once been. I reminded myself that they were far more than my parents. They were human, trying to figure out how to navigate life just the same as me. And they had made mistakes, just as I had. I wanted a chance at a different relationship, even if it happened in the slowest steps imaginable.

They arrived and I began the practice of breathing deeply before responding to them, trying to rewire my reactions. We went for walks with my dad, laughing and joking with an ease I had been missing since I was a kid. Tyler cooked chicken tacos with my mom, trying to form a connection and get to know her. I observed, wondering if I would get to know her someday, too. As we all sat at the dinner table in the home I had attempted to create with Jon,[*] I couldn't help but notice how much had already changed. I wondered if it was me or if my parents were changing too. I was able to relax my shoulders just a little as we talked about the possibility of bringing them to Washington to see Mount Rainier up close. I had done so much to keep them far away from my life in the mountains, but with Tyler's gentle support, I was starting to feel more open to letting them in. They were no longer my only family. I had this now, and I could create new bonds that would help heal the missing spaces. I didn't need them to be anything for me now. I could see them as they were and we could have a chance to move forward. Tyler coached me into the idea that I could form a new relationship with my mother, reminding me that she likely was only trying her best, even if it had failed me. "She is like you—imperfect," he said sweetly, reminding me that forgiving myself could teach me how to forgive others, too. His words didn't feel like a comparison as much as an invitation to see my own pain differently. He was the softer, gentler person I aspired to be, and I studied him, aware now of the strength in that gentleness.

All those moments and days would take us to a type of growth that can only happen once you have opened all the way up. To heal, you have to break fully open. But you don't have to stay broken. I knew that I had manifested him on that mountain in July. I knew that timing was everything, and this was our time. He unpeeled layer after layer of protection and cradled it just as gently as the Green Tara had. I was untethered to the person I had spent years curating as I finally allowed myself to just be.

---

[*] Jon and I had agreed to share time at the house since I was gone most of the time. When I needed to come home, he would leave for a few weeks. We had placed it on the market but until it sold, we traded turns. Over the winter, I finally moved completely out and into a one-room cabin in a remote town an hour away. Tyler and I shared the winter there, with no internet or entertainment beyond just existing together.

20.

ALL THAT GLITTERS

2016: Tibet, China

The day was ordinary, and somehow not like any other. It was time to see if I could do it. Could I visit the highest point on Earth without oxygen? I had tried in one form or another four of the previous seasons, and here I was again. Once I left Base Camp, the days blended and there was no tidy break between night and day: There was just the clock. Watch the clock, count the hours, and quickly forget what they mean. Move slowly, but move. Breathe. Think. Don't think too much. Look up, but don't look too far up. Climb to the next camp, rest, acclimatize, go back to Base Camp, rest, and move back up, higher each time. I had calculated the time I thought it would take to climb from our 23,000-foot-high camp at the North Col* to the little green tent

---

* The first high camp on the north side of Everest in Tibet. From here I could glance down the steep face to the west and into Nepal—seeing the route I had spent the past eight seasons getting to know.

perched awkwardly on the slope 1,200 feet above, now that we were fully acclimatized and on our summit push. Tyler was my partner in life and my climbing partner, and together we had made the journey to that little green tent twice in the past two weeks. But I hadn't yet made it any higher.

I had arrived for the season in late April, armed with a new sense of honesty and Ueli's words of encouragement. The previous fall, as I was exploring the new love with Tyler and working hard on the love I had for so long been withholding from myself, I had asked Ueli if he thought I should return to Everest again. I felt unsure how Everest fit into this new life, as I had started to be honest about the reasons why I wanted so badly to climb without oxygen. I had been looking for approval and validation because I was missing it so deeply inside myself. But now, as I was doing the work to heal, I asked myself if I still felt pulled toward my goal of trying to climb without oxygen. When I asked Ueli what he thought, he was clear: "No, you have to do it. Then you move on. It won't go away until it is done."

He was right. The reasons I wanted to pursue this challenge weren't one-dimensional. It went beyond just proving myself. There was my genuine love of the mountains and the challenge they provided. I needed to pursue the curiosity of *if* I could do this. So much about the journey behind me had been about the stoic, solo quest for achievement that would be mine and mine alone. I wouldn't accept the help of oxygen or any other person. But that position had meant that, so far, the goal had remained elusive to me. Now I was working to accept that help didn't make me weak, and that asking for it was actually the bravest thing I could do.

"Do you think I can do it?" I asked Ueli. I let him see my uncertainty, now that he had given me permission to keep my dream.

"You need perfect conditions," he said, ever the practical Swiss. I had been asking if he thought I had it in me, but he answered with the basic facts. "You can't take any oxygen with you, or you will use it. And you must set a time you won't turn around before. Otherwise, you will turn around too soon, being worried about the clock. You can do it. Just do it!" He made it sound possible, not for just anyone, but for me. I planted his words in my heart like little seeds and promised myself I would tend that garden regularly. Just before I left him, he looked me in the eye and said, "Just know why you are doing it, okay? Be able to answer that." I nodded and hugged him. I remembered him telling me he climbed all of his climbs for love. I finally understood what he meant.

My original plan had been to get to 26,000 feet, the start of the high and unforgiving "death zone," giving my body a chance to adapt to that elevation before trying to summit. But on the morning of my last attempt to reach it, I woke to slow and sludgy movements, my body tired and heavy and my mind foggy. The simple task of putting on crampons took five times as long as normal. I put them on the wrong feet, a thing I hadn't done since my novice days of climbing.

"Here, let me help you." Tyler knelt next to me and gracefully unstrapped the crampons. "What do you think about taking today as another rest day?"

His suggestions were gentle and didn't feel cloaked in judgment. But I was well practiced at being hard on myself, and when he suggested he do the carry solo, I lost control of my emotions. I ripped the crampons off my feet and threw them into the snow outside of the tent door. Tears poured from my eyes. I didn't want to cry and sacrifice the precious hydration I knew my body needed to survive, but I couldn't control it. The levee on my self-consciousness splintered, and out poured days, weeks, and years of uncertainty. *I am so weak . . . why do I think I can do this? I am not good enough. I don't deserve to be here. This season will go just like every season before, failure wrapped in the clothes of success.* People said they had more respect for those who turned around, but I knew it wasn't true.

I buried my head in my hands and shuffled back into the tent as Tyler moved out. We quickly agreed that he would do a carry to the higher camp, leaving equipment there for the summit push. I would stay behind and rest.

"It is completely okay to have a bad day." He nearly whispered his words, making sure that I didn't feel judged. He knew me well enough at this point to know that appearing weak was one of my triggers; for me to be okay showing that side to him meant I truly trusted him. He cradled me with his calm tone.

I nodded and shrank into the corner of the tent among the sleeping bags, down suits, and fuel canisters. I wanted to scream at him that he didn't know what he was talking about, that I had been at this altitude before—he hadn't. I wanted to assert my experience to justify my failure. I wanted to tell him that he didn't know what it was like to have people expecting you to fail, wanting you to fail. He didn't know what it was like to be the weakest link. To want something, work so hard for something, and foolishly believe that something can be yours only to have your mediocrity continuously prove you wrong.* I wanted to open up and accept help and then have everything feel easy, but it didn't. The frustration made me want to give up—give up trying to be vulnerable and trying to do this very hard climb. I wanted to retreat to a protective place.

Instead, I resisted. I said nothing and curled into a smaller ball, listening as his crampons crunched farther away from the tent.

This was the second time on this trip I had been too weak to do a carry. The first was on our initial climb from Advanced Base Camp up to the 23,000-foot camp at the North Col just a week earlier. We each shouldered a pack weighing seventy pounds, full of our food, fuel, and Tyler's four oxygen tanks, each weighing eight pounds. We had decided not to hire any staff but instead to share Advanced Base Camp with a group of machismo Chileans who had hired Tshering Dorje. By then, Tshering had been to the top of Everest with me three times, and joined me on trek after trek in the intervening years. He had dark and earnest eyes that beamed warm kindness, and a round belly that betrayed his

---

* But he does know these feelings. We all know. Because no matter how unique I want my feelings to be, humans have grappled with these feelings forever.

strength. As a former monk, he would often chant breathy Tibetan prayers as he sat or walked. I knew his daughters, two beautiful teenage girls who shared his same shy politeness, and his wife, who spoke little English but gave very strong hugs. Tshering was a friend, and knowing that he was there felt good. He was quick to forget my failures and kind to me on my hardest days up high.

Shortly after we left Base Camp, I knew today was not my day. After an hour of walking through the rocky moraine that leads to the icy glacier above, I could feel my throat burning. The dry air in Tibet was much more brutal than just over the border in Nepal. The microdust coated the inside of my throat, making a constant tickle, which I felt starting to turn into the itchy burn that precedes a persistent cough that won't heal in the high-altitude air. I told Tyler I didn't think I should continue; I was worried I was going to burn out my throat too soon. He was supportive but annoyed at our lack of progress; we had only made it halfway to the camp where we would drop the loads we were carrying. We shuffled some things between us, with him still committed to getting up there. I gave him some essential items and watched as he shouldered an even heavier pack now. He was so graceful and so silent.

I was grateful for him as my partner. I was grateful for his lack of judgment and his strong silence. I hated showing weakness in front of him, but I was trying to soften the side of myself that said I always had to be strong, tough, or right. I was deep in the practice of letting honesty lead, even if my delicate ego didn't think it made me look good.

As though the universe wanted to further test my intentions, up strolled the Chileans with their team of four porters and tiny packs on their backs. They leered at me, getting ready to head back to Base Camp, having failed to reach my destination. Ahead they could see Tyler with a huge load, carrying more than his fair share. They didn't have to say anything—I knew. They were sizing me up, writing my story and knowing the outcome. The leader passed me slowly, "*Hola—muy suerte* you have a strong partner, *sí?*" He nodded up the hill at Tyler. I heard the unspoken words threaded through his question: *Lucky you have someone to do all the work for you.* I smiled, nodded, and shouldered my pack to descend.

I made it to the North Col on the next trip, but now, tucked into the tent at 23,000 feet with Tyler once again soldiering forward without me, I felt like a failure. In this moment I was finding it easier to be mean to myself than kind. My mind flooded with all my failures before this, reinforcing how incapable I was, how little I could do. It was all privilege and luck. I didn't earn any of it. Tears came from my eyes as I peeked out the back door of the tent to see Tyler halfway up the face toward the little green tent. He deserved this, not me. I didn't even deserve him. As my self-loathing and insecurity threatened to drown me, the little beep of the sat phone crashed my pity party. It was a text from Ueli, who was a hundred miles away on Shishapangma. *How's it going? Windy here, we go down.*

It's calm here, I am at the North Col, I texted back, catching my tears and pulling myself out of the pit of despair.

Rest up, be the Tiger, he wrote back.

I remembered what he had said to me months earlier when I had asked him whether I should come back to Everest: *Know why you are doing this.* I wasn't doing this to be the strongest load carrier. I wasn't proving anything to Tyler about my endurance or strength or stoicism. It was the opposite. I was there to be vulnerable. I was there to open myself up all the way and ask curiously what my limits were, my own honest limits in nature. I was there to show my weaknesses instead of hiding them. Ueli might have told me to be the tiger, but I read into his simple words: *Be the tiger kitten. Be an animal who is still growing. Be vulnerable. And listen to Nature, don't try to talk over her.* I pulled my headband over my eyes and drifted into a high-altitude nap, remembering that sometimes doing nothing is the best thing we can do.

Tyler dropped our gear in the tent upon his return. I thanked him for helping me and he scooted the conversation right past my weakness and made me smile. "You're cute all wrapped up in that giant sleeping bag." He kissed my cheek and I remembered that I didn't have to be perfect to be loved. We descended together to Base Camp to take our final rest before the summit push.

In the final days of rest at our shared Advanced Base Camp,* I tucked myself into my tent for long stretches of the day, beginning the mental process of readying myself for what was ahead. I listened to music, mostly Ani DiFranco, reminding me that I was strong and that I came from a long lineage of shared XX chromosomes. It was my job to honor their sacrifice by being as courageous as possible.

I read books, trying to fill the empty corners of my mind with inspiration to crowd out any possibility of doubt. I read *Alone on the Ice*, David Roberts's story of Douglas Mawson, who attempted to get to the South Pole in 1913. This book served a specific purpose on my climb. If moving my body uphill slowly while depriving myself of sleep, food, and oxygen began to feel futile or too torturous, I would visit Mawson in my mind.† I would play the mental game of "It's better than . . ."

---

* We were only kind of sharing. After that first carry the Chileans did to the North Col, they had decided to retreat to the 17,000-foot Base Camp and wait for their porters and Sherpas to carry all their loads up and get them in position for the summit. They wouldn't rely on acclimatization as much as extra oxygen, supplied and carried by Tshering and his team. Their exit from our shared camp was welcome in almost every way. Almost. They took with them three things that we had been counting on sharing— the satellite internet modem, all the meat, and the cook, Deepak. Deepak had been with me on many expeditions, and he not only managed to handle raw chicken without contaminating me or anyone else (a real miracle if you watched him fling that thing around in the tent-turned-kitchen while touching every surface in reach with slightly bloodied hands) but was a joyful human to have around. He had the build and temperament of Timon from *The Lion King*, with a smile just as big. When the Chileans left, they took him and all the tasty, savory food, and we were left with Tshering, his four staff, and a bunch of plain white rice.

† Curiously, I chose Mawson to propel me rather than his more notable counterpart, Shackleton. Shackleton did it for fame, and he got it. It corroded his sense of why he was there, and the competition killed him (albeit of a heart attack, perhaps the universe's unceremonious way of taking a person who craved ceremony). Almost no one knows of Mawson or his incredible feats of survival, and I chose him as my partner. Shackleton was Peter Whittaker. Mawson was me.

when things got tough. *It's better than peeling the soles of your feet off after forty continuous days of walking in the Antarctic cold without taking your boots off. It's better than having to eat your sled dogs because your other sled full of food, and the partner who was hauling it, disappeared into a deep crevasse. It's better than missing your boat by only a few days—the boat that would take you back home to your wife and much fanfare instead of having to spend another winter on the empty Antarctic ice sheet with a slim crew who were slowly turning on one another.* No matter how hard the days ahead became, I would never know the trials of Mawson. But I would know the motivation. We would share intent. We would be partners on a journey of insatiable curiosity about ourselves and nature and how adventure was the thread of knowledge between the two.

I nestled myself into the story as I counted out my snacks and socks. I took little breaks from packing to cuddle up with Tyler and watch old *Chopped* episodes downloaded on our computer.* I was intentional and calculating in every item. I chose the hat I liked best. I secured my gloves and my mittens together. I placed one cup of dehydrated mashed potatoes and a few slices of precooked bacon in a bag—summit fuel. Ueli had told me just to drink on the summit push and don't worry about food. I had trained the previous year by exercising intensely while fasting for twenty-four hours. I felt confident in my ability to do this. I knew I could go without food, without sleep, but one question still had no answer. I could deprive myself of basic needs and still survive. But could I go without supplemental oxygen? Could I remove the very gas of life and still survive? Could I adapt to the most minimal resources? I pushed the questions away, replacing them with another session of "It's better than . . ." *It's better than falling in a crevasse alone and trying to acrobat your way out. It's better than failing. It's better than failing to even try.*

We planned to take four days to get from the 23,000-foot North Col

---

* Horrible idea, watching cooking shows while you are at 22,000 feet on an icy glacier with no fresh food for fifty days.

camp to the top and back down to the Advanced Base Camp.* On the first day we would move from the North Col up to the little green tent where we had stored some food, our sleeping bags, and Tyler's oxygen. Day two, we would start intentionally late from the green tent to try to time our arrival at the highest camp with sunset. I didn't want to sleep at that highest high camp, I just wanted a few hours to rest and keep moving. I had attempted to do this same style of "no sleep, just rest" on my failed 2010 climb of Everest without oxygen. It was Dave Morton's idea, and it made sense. Without oxygen, minutes were more depleting than sleep was replenishing, so you minimize time out as a priority; rest could come later. We would plan to get to the highest camp with enough time for water, a bite of food, and a change of socks.†

The climb would continue on the third day, our movement knitting one day into the other so we would no longer be able to tell them apart. We planned to climb as high as we could, hopefully to the summit, and then return down, passing that torturous 27,000-foot camp, and get back to our sleeping bags at the green tent. If everything was going well, maybe we could even get down to the North Col. And on the fourth day we would make our way down to Advanced Base Camp.‡

That was the plan. Move, nearly continuously, for four days. I was going to focus on everything I knew and open myself to everything that was left to learn. Four days of curiosity would give birth to the answers I had spent a lifetime of growth and pain trying to learn.

---

* The camps on the north side are ridiculously confusing, even for someone who has been there. There is 17,000-foot Base Camp, 18,900-foot Interim Camp, 21,500-foot Advanced Base Camp, 23,000-foot North Col (maybe you could call that Camp One or Camp Two). Then you have a mix of camps spread between 24,500 and 26,000 feet, and the last camp, Camp Nine Million at this point, is at 27,000 feet.

† Those three tasks would take about three hours at almost twenty-seven thousand feet without oxygen. Think about that.

‡ A shockingly naive goal considering all that I knew from my years of time spent above 26,000 feet.

* * *

On day one, our climb back up to the North Col was unremarkable in almost every way, except for the uncertain breath-holding expectation that this was our summit push. We had read the weather forecasts, spoken with the other teams, and determined our plan. We had worked out a strategy with Tshering to summit the same day as he and his team so that we could share resources. I didn't want to admit it, but I needed to know that Tshering was there in case anything went wrong. Tyler had never climbed above 24,000 feet, and he had never used an oxygen mask. And I didn't know this route; part of the appeal of going to the north side came from the unknown. This wasn't me showing Tyler a place I knew well; we were both discovering it together, creating a new reality instead of replaying the same one I had been trapped in for years.

I had felt a very specific feeling on every other Everest summit climb, the feeling of being part of the dimensions of a universe that is big, unknown, and unspoken. As I climbed higher and the atmosphere got thinner, I felt like another world opened to me. The air was full of energy and life, like it was the place where all the souls were hanging out, waiting for their next earthly assignment. It wasn't ominous or morose or scary. It was buoyant and humble and like being a guest in your future home. Now, I began to feel this sense of universal presence around me as we moved up to the North Col on the summit push. It reassured me to know I was moving toward a familiar space. A space where I belonged.

Starting a summit push is no guarantee. You can get a weather update that holds you down, or you can arrive and find too many teams with the same plan and be forced into a wait. You can have a single bad day or five in a row. But the clock is ticking. Everest lowers her drawbridge for a brief moment each season. The little sliver of time between the 200-mile-per-hour wind and the warm, wet slurry of the impending monsoon is your only chance. The sliver is even slimmer if you are hoping to climb without oxygen. You will be slow, so you need the weather window to be big enough to allow for a caterpillar pace. You will be cold, deprived of the oxygen that floods your extremities with warm blood, so you need the day to be as warm as possible. And you need all those universal energies to align and let you through. You need permission to be there, but you can't ask for it.

As we arrived at the North Col, I felt the permission granted to me. I felt serene. This was day one, the easiest day, the shortest day. Everything after day one could go wrong. But something about this day one felt different. I could feel it in my bones. It felt like all the life I hadn't yet lived was boiling to the top and seeping out, energizing my every moment. I was hopeful, but I tamped down my optimism with practicality. We made ice into water and I drank as much as my belly would allow. We ate noodles, precooked bacon, and snacks, and reorganized our socks and mittens. I showed Tyler the oxygen mask one more time and reviewed what to do if the exhalation valve started to freeze. We went to sleep. I fell quickly into a deeply restful state and dreamed of clouds rising all around me, begging me to hop on.

I woke up in the morning to light wind and the sun hitting the outside of the tent. It was day two—time to go. With swift and practiced grace, I filled my small backpack with the few items I would need. I put on my boots and my crampons as I bit the corner of my cheek to quell the excitement that was rising from within me. Today we would move to the green tent. It wouldn't be a big day, but it would be an important one. We left the North Col behind and moved toward the steep slopes above. Tshering Dorje was moving up with his clients as well, and he was out securing each of their oxygen masks. As we started up the slope toward the green tent, Tshering yelled to me, "Didi, wait!" He shuffled up as quickly as one can in the extremely thin air of 23,000 feet. "Can you give Paldon this camera?" He handed me a little silver point-and-shoot and motioned to one of the Sherpas who was working with him, who was high above me. As I said yes, he added, "What happened to you, Didi? You are so fast now!" He said this with a genuine curiosity of his own.

I smiled and breathed deeply, begging all the oxygen to come into my body. "I am ready," I said simply, turning to continue my climb uphill. The day was warm and calm, and as the winds were coming from the south, the flank of Everest herself was protecting us from them. We climbed up and up and eventually came upon the green tent, still perched on an awkward slope. It had been mostly used as gear storage for Tshering and another team and was uncomfortable at best. But I wasn't here for comfort. The green tent was part of the practice of not needing things to be perfect. It was a practice of being grateful. We didn't have to carry this tent up or take it down, and for that I was incredibly grateful. We repeated our ritual from the night before in the late-afternoon light: eat, drink, rest.

As the morning sky cast the first light on the mountain at the start of our third day, we peeked out from the little ledge. The wind was back, and it was creating a swirling ground blizzard outside, burying the fixed lines and making the sky the dull gray of late January on a coast. This was forecasted. We knew it was going to be stormy, but we had to move up to take advantage of tomorrow—the calmest and warmest day of the year, even if that meant minus thirty degrees Fahrenheit, so cold that your breath freezes in an icicle as you exhale it. But that was as warm as it was going to be, and we had accepted this news joyously.

We departed the little green tent, heading for new ground. I asked Tyler if I could lead and set a pace that I could keep all day. He agreed and reminded me not to go too fast, which felt funny because of how slow we were moving. We had twelve hours to climb two thousand feet. With oxygen masks, this task could take us as little as three hours, but without them, the pace would be sludgy and slow. Step, rest. Breathe, breathe, breathe, breathe, breathe, breathe. Step, rest. Breathe, breathe, breathe, breathe, breathe. Each step would take between thirty seconds to a minute to transition into the next. For twelve hours. I found a sort of rhythmic meditation as we moved higher. We passed the highest tents on the tilted football-field-size expanse of the camp and traversed the rocky terrain above. The ground blizzards continued, with wind causing the fresh snow on the ground to fly up in a cyclone and obstruct our view, but we dug the ropes out, shaking free the light and sugary snow. As the sun rose in the sky, still obstructed by the clouds, the cold air turned hot and suffocating. I removed the top of my down suit, tying it around my waist in the same way I had with my jacket in kindergarten. I thought about kindergarten and wanting to run away in the red convertible with my sister. My life hadn't been what I thought it might be, but here I was. The unruly pigtails of my youth had been tamed behind a colorful cloth headband, but the unruly dreams of adventure remained.

I carried nothing except a small first-aid kit tucked into the pocket of my down suit and a tiny water bottle in another pocket. Tyler carried the things I would need for the summit climb: my food, my mittens, my goggles, and hand warmers. And he also carried two oxygen bottles of his own, and all his things. He was my hero. My love. My support. I had lived my whole life pushing people like him far away, intent on doing it myself. But this was different. We were different, and I welcomed his support in a way that only true partnership allows. We moved in tandem up, up, up. The heat turned cold as the wind switched directions and challenged us again. My pace was slowing even further, and I wondered how far above us the high camp, at 27,000 feet, was. The slope wasn't steep or persistent, but instead a gradual uphill with small rocky protrusions that seemed to take all my energy to climb over. I wondered what time it was. I didn't want to let the clock worry me. Tyler would watch the clock, the weather, and me. He would do all the things I couldn't, and we would move in such a perfect rhythm that it would be as though we were one person. He would breathe in the oxygen and exhale onto me as encouragement to keep going. I extended my neck, letting my ponytail touch my shoulders. The clouds were clearing and just above I could see the colorful dots of a camp. Tyler told me it was almost seven. It had taken us twelve hours to get here, just like I thought it would. We were on schedule. And though that wasn't impressive in any way at all, it offered me a level of contentment. I had set my goal, turned off my mind, and moved persistently toward that goal. And now here I was, almost seven hundred feet higher than I had ever been without the use of oxygen, nearly seven hundred feet higher than the point where I had slipped on the mask in 2010, in the little yellow tent with Dave. But I was a lifetime past that moment. Everything had changed in the past six years. I had changed. My throat tightened as a well of emotions rose. I wasn't too weak. I wasn't too slow. I could do this. I knew it, for the first time, in my soul.

It was ten p.m. on May 22 and we were at 27,000 feet on the north side of Mount Everest. Everything that had happened in my life up to this point had led to this moment: I was moving forward together as one with a true partner. The stakes were life and death. The obligation to respect the risks contained our survival and our success. Tucked into the tent at the highest camp, as I changed my socks and Tyler boiled water, I cried tears of gratitude that he was here, willing to do all this for me. I had never let someone help me so much. There was nothing to hide, no façade to maintain. He saw me as I was, imperfections and scars and striving and all. And for the first time in any partnership in my life, I knew I didn't have to be anything other than myself, that was enough. I was enough. We could do anything.

It was time to go. I strapped my crampons back onto my boots and attached a rubber-insulated mask over my face. It would create a little reservoir of warm air and keep my breath from freezing to my face. I had Tyler check my harness and my crampons and we set off. I wouldn't worry about the time. I wouldn't worry about what was ahead or below. I would just move.

The first hours sped by as we moved deliberately and slowly. The summit climb on the north side of Everest starts from the high camp with a long and arduous traverse for hours before you gain any elevation. We were able, surprisingly, to pass other climbers who were using oxygen. The night rotated by, marked by the movement of the stars high above my head. I fell into a practice that I had used when running. A mile of gratitude. During a hard run, I would dedicate a mile to one person or situation and spend the entire mile thinking of all that there was to appreciate. I was deep in this practice now. I was thankful for Mike having faith enough to ask me to come to Everest my first time. I was thankful for Dave Morton, who had taught me so much about climbing at high altitudes. I was thankful for Ueli, who was somewhere on a peak nearby. And I was thankful for Tyler, who was doing everything he could to make my dream happen.

The sky began to brighten, and I finally looked ahead to see how far we had to go. I didn't want to start to do the math of time, but I also wanted to know if we were going to have any chance. If it was getting light, it must be around four thirty a.m. We had been moving for six hours. It was cold, the coldest time of the day before the sun would hit us and offer some reprieve. We were still on the traverse, below the treacherous first and second steps and the fixed ladders we would use to climb over the final vertical rock before accessing the summit ridge. That meant that we had only climbed a thousand vertical feet in six hours.

My fingers felt cold and tingly, and I wiggled them to try to force the warm blood to the very tips. Was I too cold? Was I too slow? My breathing increased as I started to wonder if this was possible. Tyler stopped and turned to ask me what was wrong from behind his oxygen mask. "My . . ." *Breath. Breath. Breath.* ". . . hands." I held up my limp fingers, wrapped in a down glove and surrounded by a down mitten. He offered me another handwarmer and I held out my glove so he could shove the warm chemical pack in. I breathed and tried to even out my heartbeat and my mind. As I tried to wiggle my fingers inside my mitten, I couldn't. The new handwarmer was too big and my fingers were stuck. I panicked. "Get it out. Get it OUT!" I yelled as tears nipped my eyes. My alarm caused him to rush and ask me if it was too hot. I continued my toddler tantrum. "It's too much. It's too much. I need to turn around," I said through sobs.

Tyler looked at me with his crystal-blue eyes, as calm as the Caribbean on a summer day. "You are doing great. We are doing great. You got this. The sun is going to come up soon and everything will be better. You got this. Let's go, we got this."

I breathed deeply into his words. In doing so, I felt the embrace of his partnership. Being alone meant I would never feel the kind of support he was showing me now. And I needed it. I needed him, and he was right: Together, we were going to do this.

I shuffled my feet even more slowly forward. "You got this," I repeated to myself, again and again until the sun hit my shoulders and I started to believe it was true. Across the traverse, up the ladder of the second step and through the gully of the third step, breathe, breathe, breathe, breathe, breathe. The same thing, over and over. Again, and again. The very poetry of life is distilled to the simplest action. Breathe, move, be, breathe. I raised my eyes to see the final slope, rising to the summit. Tshering was on top, cheering and yelling and raising his arms in excitement to see us arriving. Step, breathe, breathe, breathe, breathe. Nothing more above, everything below. I stepped the final steps onto the top and fell into the embrace of first Tshering and then Tyler. I had made it.

I was halfway to my goal, with the entire dangerous and challenging descent in front of me. I felt like celebrating but I knew the hardest part was still ahead. Another American woman, Francys Arsentiev, had been here without oxygen, with her husband, on nearly this exact day eighteen years before. She, too, made it halfway. And then on the descent she became exhausted and ultimately died. Her husband also died, trying to come to her rescue. I didn't want my story to sit alongside hers.

We quickly took photos, and I made a satellite phone call to Christine, thanking her for believing in me all these years and receiving so many dire phone calls that preceded this celebratory one. Then we began our descent. It was noon. It had taken us fourteen hours to climb two thousand feet. But really, it had taken me eight years to climb two thousand feet. Or more accurately, it had taken me thirty-two years to climb two thousand feet. It had taken the three failed attempts and five summits. It had taken the death of Chhewang and the death of my marriage.

It had taken leaving my parents' home as a teenager and coming back as an adult. It had taken pushing love away and seeing the acceptance of it as weakness and then discovering that receiving love required the greatest strength. It took infidelity and living inside lies that I let define me, and then being born into who I really was. Unmasked and accepted. It took all of that to get halfway. To get to the summit required an entire lifetime of success and failure and ecstasy and pain. But to get back down would require believing that it was all worth it—that every step before was essential to arriving. I was changed and I was as vulnerable to nature as was possible, but I didn't feel scared. I felt strong and worthy of this. Tyler started descending ahead of me, pausing after a few steps and turning back. He dropped his oxygen mask so I could see his face and he said, "Will you marry me?" I nodded yes, and smiled at him, reaching for his hand. We had talked about this before, but now it was real. We would continue this climb, and this life, as us, moving as one.

The descent is always the most dangerous part of any climb, but especially this one. It had been days since I had truly slept, and I was tired and oxygen-deprived. Small errors add up quickly and equal the weight of your demise. We made our way down amid other climbers, all with oxygen. We waited our turn to rappel down the first and second steps. I noticed the sky starting to turn to the pink evening glow as we approached the high camp, and I asked Tyler what he thought we should do. We didn't have a tent here—we had borrowed a space the night before. We didn't have sleeping bags or food, and I didn't want to stay this high for another night without oxygen. But with the dark came the wind. We weighed the options and decided we would have to stay; it didn't make sense to continue. It could take us another six hours to get to our next tent. Tshering made space for us in a tent that wasn't being used and we crawled in, committed to staying as warm and as alive as possible through the night. We wouldn't sleep, too afraid that we might forget to breathe and not wake up.

At the first light, we gathered ourselves slowly to move downhill. It was snowing and the wind was making it impossible to see through the ground blizzards, but we had to move. I drank some water and willed myself out of the tent at an impossibly slow pace. I had shivered my way through the night with only my down suit to keep me warm and Tyler constantly asking if I was okay. I was, but I was depleted. As we moved downhill, the storm moved through and climbing got easier, though still treacherously slow. This was the hardest day of my life. The desire to sit down and give up fought my will to continue for the entire day. I knew I was pushing the limits of my human container. I hadn't peed in two days. I couldn't fathom eating anything. I just kept telling myself to keep moving, even if it was painfully slow. And I did.

Tyler collected our things as we descended past the North Col. I put my pack back on, but it only slowed me further and I ended up handing off nearly everything to an already overloaded and exhausted Tyler. His pack now weighed more than eighty pounds, but he kept going and kept me going. We had to get to Advanced Base Camp down at 22,000 feet. Once we were there, we would be mostly safe. The air was thicker, and we could sleep and eat and drink. Tshering was there, and Deepak, the cook, was back with hot juice and cold water.

At nine o'clock that night, I stumbled my way into Advanced Base Camp, seventeen hours after we had started that morning. I couldn't drink water or juice; I couldn't eat anything. My stomach felt like it was stuck to itself. I forced a sip of tea and crawled into the tent, taking off my boots for the first time in two and a half days. My toes felt tingly and asleep, but they looked okay. I shed my long underwear and crawled into the yoga pants that I had kept for this very occasion. I fell into a fitful sleep, wrapped up in wisps and swaths of oxygen.

I woke up the next morning with my face swollen from the altitude and exertion. I knew it was going to take some time to physically recover from the arduous descent, but I couldn't believe how depleted I felt. I took off my socks and reexamined my feet. One small blister on my right pinky toe, and my right big toe was either bruised or frostbitten. I couldn't tell yet, but Tyler and I shared tingly numb fingers and toes—a sign that at minimum we had frost-nipped our extremities. I made my way to the dining tent and tried to eat a piece of bread and drink some water. I still hadn't peed, and eating the dry bread made my stomach spasm and my throat gag. I told Tyler I didn't think I could walk the fourteen miles it would take to get us to Base Camp without another day of rest. He agreed and we lounged about for the remainder of the day, periodically finding the energy to pack an item into our duffels that would ride on yaks across the rocky moraine to Base Camp. He must be exhausted, I thought, as I tried to muster the energy to shove my sleeping bag into a duffel. He had done so much; he had been so hardworking and selfless for my dream. And he was still carrying an unfair amount of the weight. I would find a way to thank him, but not today. In the morning we made our way to Base Camp, fourteen miles below the Advanced Base Camp over challenging terrain. We did it. We descended into a life that was full and waiting for us, bringing with us an experience that nothing could take away.

EPILOGUE

July 2021: Washington State

It is okay if you can't make it, we can figure something else out. I typed the words onto the dirty screen of my iPhone and hit send, not sure what I was hoping would happen. I felt the little flush of adrenaline as it flowed from my heart down to my legs. This was a long time coming, and a very big part of me hoped it would work out. The other part of me hoped it wouldn't.

Lhakpa responded back quickly. *No problem sister, I will make it work. See you soon.* And with that, I exhaled. It was time. It was past time. In just two days I would be on a mountain with Lhakpa Tenzing Sherpa. It had been ten years since his father, Chhewang, had died. It had been ten years since his father's death while climbing with me. It had been ten years since I felt this scared. Heading into the mountains with Lhakpa filled me with the nervous unknown of something I hoped would go well but, as life had shown me again and again, might not.

Much had changed in the past ten years . . . I had changed in that time, and, of course, so had he.

Lhakpa was twenty-one now and a remarkable young man. He was attending college in Seattle, starting his junior year at the end of the summer. His wide smile was the same as his father's. His gentle eyes hid behind dark-rimmed glasses that seemed to always need a little nudge farther up his nose. When he spoke, his mastery of English was clear, but he still had the sweet accent of a Sherpa, raised in Nepal and nestled in tradition. I had watched him grow from a young boy into a man. He was tall and skinny and gentle, just like his father. He was quick to make a joke, just like his father. My heart ached at the notion that our connection was through the most tragic circumstance. I loved knowing Lhakpa, but I wished our relationship wasn't born with his father's death.

As the years passed, I had forced my way into the lives of Lhakpa, his older brother, Ang Gyaltsen, and their mom, Lamu Chikee. I sat through many cups of tea, uncomfortable for us all. I often questioned if what I was doing was right, if I should just stay away. But I knew that staying away wouldn't change anything and showing up just might, no matter how hard it could feel. I had survived, and now this was the business of surviving the surviving.

In the time immediately following Chhewang's death, Dave Morton and I had co-founded a nonprofit, the Juniper Fund, through which we supported the families of workers killed in the mountains with five-year cash grants, vocational training, business grants, and community programs. In the time since Chhewang's death, the fund that we started in his honor grew to support more than sixty families, all connected through a web of tragedy. Each time another death occurred, Dave and I would sit with the family, unsure if what we were doing was enough. I kept close contact with Lhakpa Tenzing, trying to listen and do the right thing. Now, ten years later, I again wondered if I was doing the right thing.

Lhakpa excelled in school in Nepal and received a scholarship and a visa to come to college in the U.S. On arrival, he became one of the most well-loved students in his class. He quickly got involved in the outdoor program at his college, and as I saw images on his social media of him rafting and skiing and rock climbing, I decided to ask him if he wanted to join me on a climb. He was living just a few hours from me, though my fear and his pain kept us confined to communicating mostly over text messages. I felt the pull deep in my heart to connect with him, and so I invited him to join me on Koma Kulshan, a glaciated peak that offers all the beauty with few of the hazards of other big mountains. He excitedly said yes, and we picked a date for him to join an existing climb that I was guiding. As soon as I offered to climb with him, I wondered if I would be brave enough to follow through. Now, just one day before the climb, it was clear that it was going to happen. There was no getting out of it. All there was left to do was show up and take it all in.

My life had changed so much in the years since Chhewang's death. Some of the biggest changes had happened in the years after I finally stood on the summit of Everest without oxygen. Tyler and I got married on the beach with our parents and siblings present. I asked my parents to come, and I opened myself to them in a way I hadn't been able to do before. I let them see me cry. I showed them who I really was, still guarding myself, but far more open and vulnerable than I had ever been before. I tried to see them for who they were, too, understanding that it might take a whole other life for that to happen, or it might not ever happen, and that was okay. The next year, as spring came again, with it came a new feeling. I didn't feel the urgent pull to go back and climb on Everest. I felt at peace not trying to ascend again, much to my surprise. I had reached my goal, and the escape that Everest had provided me for so many years was no longer what I was seeking.

But I still returned, with a smaller objective and this time with Ellie. Since she had been the one with me as I reconnected with Tyler on Rainier, we asked her to officiate our small wedding. She was now fifteen and blossoming into a teenager, and I adored seeing her continue to grow from the twelve-year-old I had shared a summit with years before. Our trip to Nepal in the spring of 2017 was liberated from the pressure of summits and the constant background noise of *Will she or won't she* I had endured for the previous eight seasons. I had done it; I had reached my goal, and now I was free to pursue the joy of the mountains in a different way.

Ueli was back on Everest, still attempting the route that brought him and Simone together in 2013, the year of the fight. We had stayed in constant contact and I had grown a deep love for him and all he had shared with me. In many ways, I knew I wouldn't be where I was without him. As Ellie and I trekked, Ueli and I shared banter and tried to plan a meetup over WhatsApp and sat phone text messages. But our timing was off, and the night that Ellie and I spent sleeping at Everest Base Camp was the same night Ueli was making a final run up high to adjust to the altitude before he was ready to try for the summit. We waited late into the next morning and, after not hearing from him, decided to head down. Maybe he would catch us, as he was fast and capable, I knew.

But he didn't catch us. Instead, when we arrived back in Namche with Lhakpa and Cherap, I was greeted with the terrible news that there was an accident. He had fallen. He was gone.

In the days that followed, I flew back to Kathmandu, tucking Ellie into a hotel with Chhewang's son Lhakpa to keep her company. I went to the Swiss embassy with Ueli's wife, Nicole, helping her in this most unmanageable time. I went to the monastery and purchased all the items for a traditional Buddhist cremation with the help of a gracious monk.

I held his death certificate in my hand while tears and anger poured out of me like a storm. I wasn't supposed to be preparing him to be cremated. I was supposed to be running in the mountains with him. He was the tiger. Not a small and lifeless body draped in white cloth and a marigold garland.

As his body was laid over the flames with Everest just in the distance, everyone cried. I filled cups of tea and made sure there was always a chair near his mother, so she could have a place to rest her body on the worst day of her life. Nicole stayed away from the others, lighting butter lamps and wiping the tears from her own eyes in private. I allowed my tears to pour out and rested my hands over my heart, trying to hold it together as I saw so many people feel the immense loss of a soul so bright. I felt so grateful that I could be here to say goodbye to him. He was the person who had shown me what it means to be yourself.

I wondered if I could be myself without him here to keep showing me the way. He had given me more than I had ever been able to tell him. You are a tiger, too, he said. And he was right. *It is better to live one day as a tiger than a thousand years as a sheep.* With his death it felt for a moment that life wouldn't continue.

But it did. And the next spring, Tyler and I welcomed our daughter, Kaia.

In the weeks after her birth, I moved effortlessly. Silently. Almost floating from one room to the next. My body had purpose. A purpose that anchored me to the very floor I walked across, but at the same time my whole being was filled with light spaciousness, as though I could just as easily float away as I could sink into the floor. My being was a seesaw of rooting and flying. It was at this moment, this incredibly ordinary but somehow also extraordinary moment, that I understood the difference between being rooted and being anchored. An anchor is a device of man, weighing you down and keeping you in a place you may have only intended to visit. Roots are the divine things of nature, meant to absorb the wisdom and nourishment from every moment and pour them through you so you can grow up and extend outward and become all of the possibilities.

As this revelation crossed my mind, I felt her little body wiggle gently against mine. She was squished impossibly tightly into the fabric wrap, pressed close to my chest and heart. She was eighteen days old and eight tiny pounds. But she was also the weight of balance. She was the equilibrium to every story that had played out prior to her arrival, and at the same moment, my arrival. There is an impossibility in knowing who you are meant to be until you become that person. Until the day you get to see yourself and recognize her to be your own home as well as your own self. The striving can stop, and the being can begin. In my case, it took my entire life to get here. It took death in my life, and the death of many versions of who I thought I was. It took conscious effort and continuous healing to become a human who could greet this new person and know that my greatest contribution to the world would not be paving a path for anyone else. It would not be in any accomplishment, and it certainly wouldn't be in any summit. It would be in sharing roots with her and allowing her to be my wings. It would be in allowing her to be my teacher. I had always imagined that becoming a mother would weaken me and soften me and make me useless. But here, on this quiet morning in my home with newborn Kaia pressed against my actual heart, it was clear. She was my reinforcement. She would soften me, and that would become my greatest strength and my greatest use. She was the possibilities. She was my roots and wings, and together we would fly.

But flying wouldn't mean that I could escape my past. And part of my journey of healing involved connecting with Lhakpa in a deeper way. So, in the early morning of a warm June in the Cascades, I met the clients and Lhakpa at the gas station below the mountain we hoped to climb. I helped him pack his gear into his backpack and handed him a set of crampons and an ice axe to borrow. I held my breath and blurred my eyes to avoid looking too hard at the ways he moved just like his father. We headed up the trail, me in front followed by the two clients and Lhakpa in the back. As we talked about things both big and small, I would hear his closed-lipped noises of acknowledgment that he was listening. He moved gracefully and knowingly up the mountain toward camp under the weight of his heavy pack. Mountaineering was new to him, but it was also deep in his bones, the little strands of DNA that connected him to his father. I said goodnight as he crawled into his one-man tent and I into mine. The nylon walls weren't enough for me to feel any sort of distance, and my mind started doing acrobatics about the climb ahead. A hot wet tear nipped at the edge of my eye at the thought that his dad should be the one showing him these mountains, not me.

My thoughts surrendered to a restless sleep until midnight, when my alarm woke me abruptly, as it had so many nights before. I sat up and looked out at the night sky. It was a new moon—my favorite type to climb under. The stars shone brilliantly in all their glory, undimmed by any light from the moon. Chhewang died on a full moon, and I had vowed to never climb on one again. It felt important that this climb with Lhakpa was under the dark sky.

There was no wind, and the air was warm. It felt right, like where I should be. We got ready in the rhythm of every climb I had done before, but this one was something different. I double-checked Lhakpa's crampons before we tied into the rope and set foot on the glacier. At the first crunch of the metal spikes pushing into the firm ice, my breath caught in my throat, refusing to budge, and forcing me to acknowledge the enormity of what I was about to do. I looked back at Lhakpa's head-lamp, shining brightly toward me and the unknown ahead. We had nothing left to do but climb, so we began.

The climbing was slow and thoughtful. We moved like a sedated snake, intentional but in no hurry. The slope of firm ice steepened as the sun ascended rhythmically over the horizon, casting its warm light on us. I yelled back to Lhakpa, forty feet away from me at the end of the rope. "You doing okay?" He smiled his big warm smile and replied, "Ya, sis, I am good." I continued forward, leading our rope as we made the final steep climb to the top. Just before the summit, I stopped. I yelled back to Lhakpa to come up to me. He fumbled with the rope as it created loops around his feet as he rushed up to my side. "Everything okay?" he asked, with a worried wrinkle in his brow. The summit was in sight, only five minutes away. "It is okay. I wanted to see if you want to lead us to the top." His deep brown eyes shone back at me as he nodded and led the rope team to the top. As I walked behind his skinny frame, my face reddened and my chest tightened. Tears came uncontrollably out of my eyes. Seeing him move with grace in the same way his father did brought me both pain and gratitude. I cried for what was lost, and now, for what was gained.

I had lost so much in the years behind me. Friends had died. Marriages had failed. My motivations for existing had changed. But I had gained far more. I had learned the fine art of acceptance, of myself and others. I had grown into a faithful wife, showing up for Tyler with joy, never even feeling the illusion of captivity. We were partners, building a life. We had a beautiful daughter and a son on the way. We had a peaceful home with two cats and so much love. What I had lost made space for all that I had gained.

At the summit, we unclipped from the rope and linked arms for the final steps to the tippy-top of the mountain. I gave Lhakpa a hug, standing on the ends of my crampons to meet his height. Despite the bright glow of the sun on the glacier, I took off my sunglasses, wanting him to see my eyes.

"Lhakpa, I am so sorry your dad couldn't show you this." My words reached his ears and immediately he started crying. I embraced him firmly in a hug and held his hands in my own. "Thank you for letting me be in your life. Thank you for being here. It means so much." We embraced and our tears pressed into each other's, creating one flow, tangled together as our lives would forever be. The simple act of getting to live another day in this complicated life would forever be *enough*. It didn't require us to hold back our tears or to be perfect people. It didn't require accomplishments or accolades. I had tried so hard to prove that I was worthy, and that journey had taken me from the darkest corners of my mind all the way to the top of the world in search of belonging. But here, on this beautiful and ordinary day, standing on the crystal white glacier with a sapphire sky above, I could see clearly that what I had scoured the Earth for had been inside of me all along.

AUTHOR'S NOTE

This memoir reflects my personal experiences and the emotions I've carried throughout my life. While I've done my best to capture the truth, memory is subjective and evolves with time. Some names, details, and identifying characteristics have been changed to protect the privacy of individuals and to provide narrative clarity. Some conversations have been recreated from memory and are not verbatim representations.

I also want to note that my mother, a central figure in some of these stories, has expressed a different perspective on the events and memories I recount here. This is my version of the story, shaped by my journey, and it is shared with the hope of shedding light on the complexities of family, memory, and self-understanding.

Ultimately, this memoir reflects my personal truth, not an absolute record of events. I invite readers to engage with it as a piece of my heart, knowing that it is, in part, shaped by the lens through which I've come to see my past.

ACKNOWLEDGMENTS

This book, like so many things in my life, would not be possible without the help, support, and love of so many people. First, I owe a huge debt of gratitude to my husband, Tyler. He has not only loved me through all of my learning, but he has loved me while I insisted on sharing all my mistakes with the world. This is no small task and it deserves a moment here of pure gratitude. Thank you, Tyler. You are all that glitters and my world wouldn't be nearly what it is without you by my side.

Kaia, my sweet daughter who has healed so many wounded parts of me, thank you, sweet girl, you are forever my guide. And Judah, my sensitive and silly boy, thank you for being the bright side of any tough situation. Thank you to my sister, Stephanie, for being my first best friend, for truly knowing all the versions of me, and for showing me love for my whole life. I wouldn't have survived the toughest years if I didn't have you, and I am so grateful to be able to call you a friend and my family. And to my dad. I was unsure of many things in my life but I was never unsure of your love for me. Thank you for loving me even when I hurt you. You were my first hero and you are still that hero today. I love you.

This book lived in my head and heart for many years but without the help and support of a few key people, it would still be there today. Chris Kriesen, thank you for persistently listening and accepting all the versions of my story until a structure emerged. I couldn't have done this without you. Adrienne Schaefer, you endured so many verbal drafts of my story and somehow stayed my friend. Thank you for all the long runs to talk through it and for loving me in the end. Christine Hass (and the whole Hass family), you are my family, and I am constantly amazed that I somehow have managed to keep you in my life—I know we are in it together, forever. Maddie Miller, you have been a friend and the little sister I never knew I needed. Thank you for being my family and loving me unconditionally. Allison Groenleer, Adam and Alice, Ben Ringe: You all took great care and kindness with early drafts and helped give me the courage to keep going. To Annelies, for holding me so closely and loving me as I showed up. To my sister-in-law, Phoebe, and my in-laws Libby and Nick, thank you for allowing me to be a part of your family, it has been such an incredible family to join. Thank you, Amber, for holding my heart as I have navigated growth, your kindness has meant so much to me. Kristen Elliott, thank you for always lifting me up and believing in me, I wouldn't have been able to do any of this without your support. A huge thank-you to so many of my amazing clients who have listened to my stories and who told me I had one worth telling—particularly Phil, JP, Juliana, Bob and Julie, Kendra, Kevin, Leslie, Sarah, Ellie, and truly anyone I have shared a rope with. Thank you, Dave Morton, for being my friend, mentor, and climbing partner. You have taught me so much. I have countless mentors and teachers from the guiding community, especially in the early days of working at RMI, who have allowed me to grow into the guide I have become. Thank you to Autumn, Lacie, and Sarah and the endlessly patient office girls who listened to my drama and held my hand as I figured out how to navigate it all. And Jeff, thank you for always letting me take the seat and say my words, it meant more than you probably knew. Thank you to Damian and Willie for being my brothers and for weaving your lives so kindly into mine. Thank you to Lary Bloom for your help and guidance. Thank you to Dr. Pasang Yangee Sherpa for reviewing my words and helping me see things more clearly. Lhakpa bai and Ang Gyaltsen bai—words will never be able to convey my gratitude that you have allowed me into your lives. An enormous thank you to Liz Parker, for being my champion and my sensei through it all. And lastly, thank you to Kevin Doughten. You saw my story through my messy words and helped me tell it, and I am forever in debt to you and the kindness you showed throughout the process.

I want to acknowledge that this book and this story wouldn't exist without the mistakes I made along the way. Being human is hard and I have hurt people as I have tried to figure it out. I am sorry to the people who were impacted by the messiness of my growth. I have tremendous gratitude that I have had a chance to grow and change and do things a little better each day. I have grown with the help of professionals who have tenderly cared for my mental health and help me stay accountable to being the person I know I can be—thank you so much for helping me. And if you are struggling to get to your own summit and the climbing feels too hard, please know that I think the journey is a worthwhile one, for us all.

About the Author

MELISSA ARNOT REID is the first American woman to summit Everest without supplemental oxygen. It was her sixth summit of the highest ground on Earth, cementing her place in mountaineering history. In doing so, she became a media star and in demand from many publications, television shows, and organizations looking for inspirational speakers. She continues to work as a mountain guide all over the world and runs the Juniper Fund, the nonprofit she cofounded.